D0050639

preventing arthritis

ALSO BY RONALD M. LAWRENCE, M.D., PH.D., AND MARTIN ZUCKER:

The Miracle of MSM: The Natural Solution for Pain
(with Stanley W. Jacob, M.D.)

ALSO BY RONALD M. LAWRENCE, M.D., PH.D.:

Magnet Therapy: The Pain Cure Alternative
(with Paul J. Rosch, M.D., and Judith Plowden)

Going the Distance: The Right Way to Exercise for People over 40
(with Sandra Rosenzweig)

Goodbye Pain!

Pain Relief with Osteomassage

ALSO BY MARTIN ZUCKER:

Natural Hormone Balance for Women (with Uzzi Reiss, M.D.)

The Veterinarians' Guide to Natural Remedies for Dogs

The Veterinarians' Guide to Natural Remedies for Cats

Pet Allergies: Remedies for an Epidemic
(with Alfred J. Plechner, DVM)

preventing

arthritis

A HOLISTIC APPROACH TO LIFE WITHOUT PAIN

Ronald M. Lawrence, M.D., Ph.D., and Martin Zucker

G. P. Putnam's Sons
New York

Every effort has been made to ensure that the information contained in this book is complete and accurate. However, neither the publisher nor the author is engaged in rendering professional advice or services to the individual reader. The ideas, procedures, and suggestions contained in this book are not intended as a substitute for consulting with your physician. All matters regarding your health require medical supervision. Neither the author nor the publisher shall be liable or responsible for any loss, injury, or damage allegedly arising from any information or suggestion in this book.

G. P. Putnam's Sons
Publishers Since 1838
a member of
Penguin Putnam Inc.
375 Hudson Street
New York, NY 10014

Published simultaneously in Canada

Photographs by Martin Zucker; model: Katie Regan

Library of Congress Cataloging-in-Publication Data

Lawrence, Ronald Melvin, date.
Preventing arthritis : a holistic approach to life without pain /
Ronald M. Lawrence and Martin Zucker.
p. cm.
Includes bibliographical references and index.
ISBN 0-399-14742-X
1. Arthritis—Popular works. 2. Arthritis—Prevention.
I. Zucker, Martin. II. Title.
RC933.L37 2001 00-068857
616.7'22—dc21

Printed in the United States of America

10 9 8 7 6 5 4 3 2 1

This book is printed on acid-free paper. ♾

Book design by Mauna Eichner

TO OUR BELOVED GRANDCHILDREN:

ALLISON AND JEREMY LYONS

JOSHUA, MAX, NOAH, NATHAN, AARON, AND RACHEL GOTTLIEB

Acknowledgments

We would like to express our gratitude to the following individuals, who shared their experience, recommendations, and insights and contributed to the enrichment of our book: Robert Ansley, Jr.; Thomas J. Bassler, M.D.; Tim Batchelder; Fereydoon Batmanghelidj, M.D.; Steve Blair, P.E.D.; David Brownstein, M.D.; Bob Delmonteque, N.D.; John M. Ellis, M.D.; Keith Gall; Lonnie Grant; Denham Harman, M.D., Ph.D.; Frederick C. Hatfield, Ph.D.; Abram Hoffer, M.D., Ph.D.; Stanley W. Jacob, M.D.; Ingrid Kelsey; Evarts Loomis, M.D.; Robert E. Markison, M.D.; Richard Markoll, M.D., Ph.D.; Larry Payne, Ph.D.; Deborah Quilter; Vivian Redman; Paul J. Rosch, M.D.; Anthony L. Rosner, Ph.D.; Susan Schiffman, Ph.D.; Benjamin Shield, Ph.D.; Artemis P. Simopoulos, M.D.; D. Edwards Smith, M.D.; Steven Subotnick, D.P.M., D.C., N.D.; Moti Tiku, M.D.; Melvyn R. Werbach, M.D.; and Marc White.

To Katie Regan, for being such a gracious off-duty model.

To Jack Scovil, a much valued agent and, once again, to Stacy Creamer, our editor, for editorial guidance.

And to Lesli Lawrence, for providing access to her beautiful garden as an inspiring meeting place for two toiling authors.

Note to the Reader

This book about arthritis prevention is not intended as medical advice and should not be used to replace medical care or any therapeutic program recommended by a physician. It is meant for information and education only.

If you have symptoms or suffer from an illness, consult with an appropriate health professional before carrying out any information presented in this book.

If you are currently taking prescription drugs, do not discontinue them or replace them on the basis of any information in the book without first consulting your doctor.

Contents

PART I
why an ounce of prevention is worth a ton

PART II
ten steps for preventing arthritis

PART III

becoming an anti-arthritis warrior

PART I

why an ounce of prevention is worth a ton

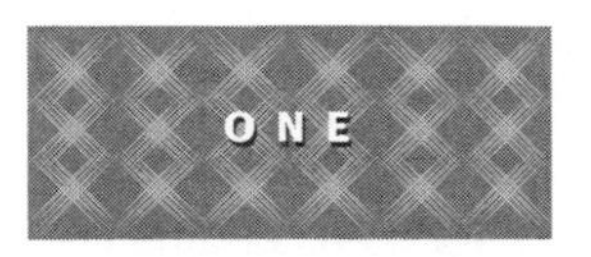

The Osteoarthritis Epidemic Ahead

- Until she developed arthritis in the knees, Sandra had always been a hefty, food-loving woman active in family and local affairs. In order to avoid pain, the seventy-two-year-old grandmother spent more time on the sofa watching TV and became increasingly inactive. Her weight soared, her pain increased, and so too did her anxiety, blood pressure, blood sugar, and dependence on others.

- Elaine, fifty-seven, a slender secretary in the entertainment industry, developed severe arthritis in the hands and lower back. Seeking relief, she went from doctor to doctor and collected multiple prescriptions for painkillers. The medication took a huge toll on her body. Besides becoming fatigued and constipated, she developed ulcers and digestive problems.

- John was an ambitious, macho colonel eyeing the rank of general. For years he had prided himself on his strength and toughness. After hitting fifty, however, he began experiencing pain, stiffness, and reduced range of motion in the knees and shoulders. The diagnosis of arthritis and growing discomfort undermined his confidence. His sex life suffered. His stress level grew. A physician prescribed cortisone for the pain. At first he felt better but soon developed bothersome side effects. He stopped the medication and refused to take any drugs. The pain and motion limitation increased, as did his stress level and depression. Unable to cope with his condition and the job, John decided to take an early retirement.

You may think that arthritis merely causes some pain and discomfort that can usually be eliminated with a pill or joint replacement and you are right back in the groove again.

You're misguided if you think so.

During fifty years in a pain practice, and having treated more than 150,000 patients, I have seen arthritis ruin the lives of many people like Sandra, Elaine, and John.

The reality is that arthritis erodes the ability to function. Lost function can prevent you from taking part in basic and cherished activities, lead to other health problems, and rob you of both quality and length of life. Unfortunately, the solutions we in the medical profession offer are much less than ideal and often the cause of additional problems.

Arthritis doesn't take out people in an instant like a heart attack or a stroke, or overrun vital organs like cancer, but it can create a domino effect of crippling, depressing, and slowly lethal consequences.

Edward H. Yellin, Ph.D., of the Rosalind Russell Medical Research Center for Arthritis at the University of California at San Francisco, puts it this way: "No condition impairs the quality of life of more older adults—and to a greater extent—than does arthritis."

Here's how:

- Arthritis promotes inactivity and disability, limiting everyday activities such as working, walking, exercising, and even dressing and bathing. The nature of life is movement, and inactivity is a ticket to heart disease, stroke, obesity, diabetes, cancer, and high blood pressure.

- Arthritis contributes to the long-term use of painkillers and anti-inflammatories, drugs that sap energy and health and have serious side effects.

- Arthritis also contributes to stress, anxiety, and depression, which in turn are major risk factors for many serious diseases and the use of medications that further deplete health.

Pain

Inactivity

Disability

Stress

Medication side effects

These are the accomplices of arthritis.

There are many different types of arthritis, but far and away the most prevalent is osteoarthritis, also known as degenerative joint disease, wear-and-tear arthritis, or just plain arthritis. The incidence increases with age and for that reason is widely regarded as part of the aging process. However, it is a common condition by middle age, and not just a disease of the elderly.

Osteoarthritis affects more than 21 million Americans, an "official" estimate by experts based on the most recent available data. But the experts—members of the National Arthritis Data Workgroup—believe their estimate is conservative and that the real incidence is much higher.

That's because arthritis is one of the most self-treated diseases, as reflected by huge sales of over-the-counter arthritis medications. Many people choose to deal with the condition without seeing a physician. Or, if they do see a physician, they may not get an X-ray confirmation of arthritis. In my own pain practice, one out of three patients sees me for arthritis-related complaints.

Whatever the real numbers now, public health agencies are sure that in the not-too-distant future the incidence is going to rise to the level of an epidemic. That prospect has officials so alarmed they have begun mobilizing national resources to confront a major health-care challenge.

"As the leading edge of the baby boom generation enters the prime years for arthritis," the Arthritis Foundation has warned, "a quantum leap will take place as the number of people affected surges and the impact on individuals and the nation's health grows dramatically."

The projection is this:

The percentage of Americans over sixty-five years of age is the most rapidly growing segment of the population. By the year 2020, with the aging of the baby boomers, an estimated 60 million people will have some form of arthritis, and well over half will involve osteoarthritis.

With an anxious eye on a looming medical crunch, the Arthritis Foundation, the Centers for Disease Control and Prevention (CDC), and the Association of State and Territorial Health Officials huddled together in 1998 and created the first comprehensive public health approach to reducing the burden of arthritis in the United States. A $10 million National Arthritis Action Plan was launched. The goal: delaying the onset of pain and disability due to arthritis among individuals by ten years and extending a more vigorous, vital life. Research indicates this is possible. One study found that people with the lowest-risk lifestyles had up to an eight-year delay of disability.

From my pain practice, I know this is possible. I have seen many patients stay free of arthritic symptoms well into their seventies and eighties by following a good lifestyle. Sometimes I gave these patients guidelines that I felt could help prevent or delay the disease. Other times they followed healthy routines on their own. In many cases, I have been able to help arthritic patients substantially minimize pain or prevent it from getting worse.

Osteoarthritis Facts

- Osteoarthritis is the most common chronic disease affecting older people.
- Almost all people over sixty-five have X-ray evidence of osteoarthritis in some joints, but many don't have symptoms.
- Pain is the primary symptom.
- Eighty percent of individuals with osteoarthritis report some degree of limitation in movement or activities.
- The condition is progressive, a process of deterioration that probably started many years before.
- Osteoarthritis can affect any of the movable joints of the body from top to bottom—the vertebrae of the spine from your neck down to your lower back, the shoulders, elbows, wrists, fingers, hips, knees, ankles, feet, and toes.
- It can, and often does, affect more than just one joint.
- Moderate to severe symptoms are almost twice as high among women, and overall two to four times more prevalent than among men.
- It has a huge effect on the burden of disability and dependence among older Americans.
- It ranks second only to heart disease as the cause of adults receiving Social Security disability payments.
- Osteoarthritis and other arthritic conditions rack up a huge toll in medical bills and productivity losses, estimated as possibly exceeding 2 percent of the gross domestic product.

how to use this book

My purpose in writing this book is to warn you not to take arthritis lightly and to offer ideas for preventing it. An ounce of prevention is worth a pound of cure, the old saying goes, but with arthritis, there is no cure. Once you've got it, you've got it and have to deal with it. That makes every ounce of prevention worth a ton. *Preventing Arthritis* is my attempt to help you personally meet—and even exceed—the declared goal of the National Arthritis Action Plan.

It can be done.

You can become an anti-arthritis warrior.

I myself, at the age of seventy-five, have managed to stay pain free by practicing much of what I preach.

And I know from clinical experience that painful, debilitating symptoms are not always inevitable even though most of us are likely to develop arthritis as we age. I also know from my patients that you can substantially slow down the progression of disease and minimize the symptoms if they develop.

There is much you can do to protect and fortify yourself.

Many of the physiological changes leading to osteoarthritis are not yet clearly understood by medical science. So prevention is an effort in which you take aim at the risk factors that contribute to joint damage. In this book, I will arm you with the guidelines to do so, the very same advice I share with my patients. In order to make the book even more effective, I have also called upon experts to share their recommendations.

Preventing Arthritis is divided into three parts. In the first part, I will give you a brief review of how osteoarthritis develops and what the major risk factors are. In chapters 3 and 4 I will cover the serious consequences of arthritis—pain, stress, inactivity and disability, medication side effects, and the increased risk of obesity and developing other diseases.

Part Two contains ten chapters—ten steps for preventing arthritis. This is the practical information to protect your joints. Some of the recommendations do not require additional time out of your day, but rather modifying how you sit, stand, walk, work, eat, and carry out everyday tasks. Other measures, such as yoga and exercise, do require time. But the time involved is well worth it.

The biggest time factor in arthritis prevention is getting enough exercise. If you presently exercise regularly for cardiovascular and fitness purposes, you are already making an important commitment to your health. Now you need to ensure that what you are doing helps, and not hurts, your joints.

In Part Two, I'll cover strategies for the well-known risk factors such as excess weight and trauma inflicted on the joints through accidents, work, and sports activities. I'll also discuss ideas that you probably have not read elsewhere about how to prevent or minimize symptoms, by, for instance, drinking enough water, or reducing (if you are a woman) your use of high heels, and how to protect your precious hands, the most common site of arthritis in the body. There may even be a role for sex in arthritis prevention, and I'll talk about that as well. And there is a chapter packed with the latest information on many effective nutritional supplements.

In Part Three, I summarize my recommendations into a quick guide to personal prevention strategy and also make recommendations for doing some very beneficial "extras" that involve professional care—acupuncture, chiropractic, massage, and Rolfing. Each of these approaches offers both preventive and therapeutic benefits. Preventively, they can potentially correct anatomical misalignments or faulty biomechanics leading to joint degeneration.

For those who have arthritis already, I have filled a chapter in part 3 with recommendations on new and natural therapy options. This information includes an exciting new noninvasive procedure called pulsed signal therapy that is soon to be approved for use in the United States. While you can't cure arthritis, there are many ways—on your own or with professional help—to slow down progression of the condition, relieve pain, and increase your overall health in the process.

With the scientific data now available, osteoarthritis can be prevented or at least minimized in many instances. There is much you can do to protect your joints from degeneration. Today, a good anti-aging program must include recommendations not just for a healthy heart, but for healthy joints as well. You may not be able to follow all the recommendations I have put in this book, but that's OK. Do what you can do. But think preventively for your joints, just as you do for your heart. Instead of learning to live with pain and disability, I say learn to prevent them! You can go the distance with healthy joints, or at least healthier joints, and you will be better off than if you do nothing and just wait for arthritis to overtake you. And by helping your joints, you'll be helping your whole body as well.

TWO

How Osteoarthritis Happens

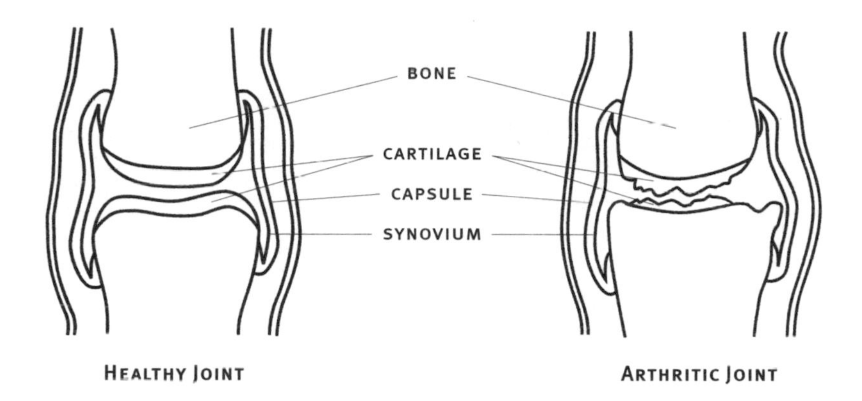

During his forty years as a pathologist at Centinela Hospital in Inglewood, California, Thomas J. Bassler, M.D., examined thousands of arthritic knees and hips that were removed from patients undergoing joint replacement surgery.

"You see basically the same diseased picture," he says. "The shiny cartilage is gone or mostly gone. Instead, there is abnormally thickened bone tissue, smooth and gray like granite, or rough and jagged like mountaintops.

"Healthy cartilage feels slick and rubbery to the touch. The exposed bone feels rough, gritty, or sandpaper-like.

"In arthritis, the joints have literally become battlegrounds, with healthy tissue blown away, and bone often painfully wearing against bone."

In understanding how to minimize the chance of your joints becoming battlegrounds—and you a casualty—we first need to start with some basics:

- What is osteoarthritis?
- How a joint works and how it becomes arthritic.
- The risk factors.

what is osteoarthritis?

osteo = bone
arth = joint
itis = inflammation

Osteoarthritis affects the joints in the body, the junctions between two or more bones that enable movement and the physical actions of life. Your knee joints, for instance, allow you to bend your legs and walk. The many joints in your hands and fingers give you the ability to grip and write.

Cartilage, the layer of tissue covering the facing surfaces of mobile joints, cushions the bones like shock absorbers and allows them to glide smoothly against or past each other. In osteoarthritis, the ability to produce or repair cartilage is unable to keep pace with the forces that damage the tissue.

A variety of causes called risk factors undermine the integrity of joints and accelerate the breakdown of cartilage. Such risk factors include injury, microtrauma from repetitive use, excess weight, or irregular forces on joints created by anatomical misalignments (see risk factors later in this chapter).

Because of various risk factors, cartilage erodes and becomes pitted over time. Degenerative changes develop in underlying bone and supporting tissue. The body tries to correct this by laying down calcium, just as you would apply Spackle to fill a hole in a wall in your house. Spikes of calcium deposits called osteophytes rise from damaged tissue and create additional problems.

The ongoing breakdown causes friction. Bones rub against bones. Low-grade inflammation develops in the membrane encapsulating the joint. When this lining swells, the liquid-filled joint space inside the capsule becomes narrower. The inflammation can also affect tendons or ligaments that help stabilize the joint.

If the risk factors are relentless, the normal repair process in the joint becomes overwhelmed. Down at the molecular level, the compounds promoting cartilage health and regeneration lose ground to the compounds promoting cartilage degradation. Moreover, as we age, the body's circulatory efficiency diminishes. Less of the essential nutrients and oxygen carried by the blood are available to feed the tissues, including the joints. Lack of exercise and poor diet aggravate this scenario.

The degenerative process has both mechanical and chemical aspects, and rather than a passive "falling to bits," it is more a case of the repairman failing to keep up with the rate of deterioration.

When cartilage deteriorates, it loses the ability to cushion the impact of major and minor shocks and trauma. A varying degree of symptoms occurs—from very mild to very severe. They include pain, tenderness, stiffness, swelling, range of motion problems, and activity limitations. As the arthritis progresses, the joints hurt with less and less activity.

Osteoarthritis vs. Rheumatoid Arthritis

Unlike osteoarthritis, rheumatoid arthritis is an autoimmune condition of an extremely inflammatory nature. Dysfunction in the immune system causes the body to attack its own tissue. The joint lining becomes chronically inflamed. Inflammation can jump like a fire from the joints to organs throughout the body, including the heart and lungs. There is pain, stiffness, and swelling in multiple joints. While not primarily a wear-and-tear process, rheumatoid causes bone and cartilage erosion and joint deformities. About two million Americans suffer with this condition, most of them women.

who's who in the joint

Joint structures differ. Some, like the vertebral bones in the spinal column are slightly moveable, while the hands, shoulders, elbows, feet, hips, and knee joints are built for wider ranges of motion.

The structures are complex. They involve variations of cartilage, supporting bone beneath the cartilage, joint capsules, and the surrounding soft-tissue support of muscles, tendons, and ligaments.

Here's a rundown of the major components in and around the joints:

Capsule

This is the sac that encases the bone ends of the joint and holds the synovial fluid. The inner lining of the sac is called the synovial membrane.

Cartilage

This soft, cushioning, bluish-white tissue covering facing bones is composed of 65 to 80 percent water, which gives the joint lubrication and wear-resistance qualities. The rest of the cartilage is collagen and proteoglycans, substances necessary for resilience, elasticity, and shock absorption. These three elements form the cartilage matrix.

Cartilage contains no blood vessels or nerves. The tissue is "fed" from the joint fluid.

In simplistic terms, think of cartilage as a sponge. When a sponge is compressed, it gives off fluid. It refills again when the pressure is released. Movement creates pressures on the joint. This results in a liquid give-and-take that facilitates mechanical shock absorption, nutrient distribution, and waste product removal.

Collagen

This structural protein accounts for 25 to 30 percent of the body's proteins and helps form tendon, skin, membranes, and bone tissues. It gives elasticity and shock-absorbing ability to cartilage. It also functions as a framework to hold proteoglycans in place.

Chondrocytes

These are primary cartilage cells that produce collagen and proteoglycan molecules. They also release enzymes that break down and remove old, unfit collagen and proteoglycan molecules.

Ligaments

These are tough tissues that attach bone to bone and provide stability for the joints. Injury or degeneration involving ligaments, muscles, and tendons can cause changes in joint mechanics and independently generate pain. Damage to the anterior cruciate ligament, for instance, often leads to arthritis in the knee joint.

Muscle

These are tissues that contract to provide the force for movement of joints as well as shock-absorbing benefits. Some muscles are attached to joint capsules. Spasm, atrophy, and weakness of muscles contribute to joint abnormalities and pain associated with osteoarthritis.

Osteophytes (Calcium Deposits)

Also known as bone spurs, these hard growths frequently form at various locations in the joint as a result of the degenerative process. They cause pain and constrict movement.

Proteoglycans

These large molecules, produced in abundance by chondrocytes, interlace with collagen fibers to build thick, resilient layers inside the cartilage tissue. They are made up of a core protein with attached chains of sugars called glycosaminoglycans (GAGs) that attract and hold water. This water-retention capacity is crucial because the water acts as a lubricant and shock absorber.

Tendons

These tough tissues attach muscles to bones, permit movement, and act as secondary joint stabilizers.

Synovium (Synovial Membrane)

This is the inner lining of the joint capsule, which secretes the thick, slippery synovial fluid. The membrane is rich in capillaries, nerves, and lymphatics. The fluid fills the space inside the capsule, providing lubrication for the joint and facilitating movement.

which joints are most affected?

Generally, osteoarthritis occurs most frequently in weight-bearing and excessively used joints. Thus, we see it most commonly in the hands, followed by the feet, then the knees and hips. The incidence in the hands, feet, and knees in almost all age groups is higher for women than men. Men tend to develop more degeneration in the cervical (neck) and lumbar spine, and the hips.

Here is what research tells us about the incidence of osteoarthritis:

The Hands

- Thirty percent of adults are estimated to have X-ray evidence of osteoarthritis. After the age of sixty-five, the incidence is 70 percent.
- The most frequent site is the basal joint of the thumb, just above the wrist.
- Gripping is a common task involving intense muscle forces on the hand joints. Men and women with the highest grip strength may be at an increased risk of arthritis in the hands.
- Older women frequently develop small, bony enlargements of the last joint of the fingers called Heberden's nodes. These growths occur in a significant number of people with osteoarthritis. There is a genetic tendency to develop this unsightly condition.

The Feet

- About 21 percent of adults, especially seniors, are estimated to have arthritis in the feet.

The Knees

- Knee osteoarthritis affects about 9.5 percent of adults over the age of sixty-two.
- Because the knees are involved in so many basic daily activities, such as walking and standing, arthritis here is a major cause of inactivity, disability, and weight gain.
- The incidence among elderly women is 1.7 times higher than among elderly men.
- Osteoarthritis is the cause of more than 70 percent of total hip and knee replacements.
- Knee arthritis may be accompanied by back pain in more than 50 percent of cases. This creates more night pain and anxiety.
- Primary risk factors are excess weight, previous knee injury, occupational knee bending, heavy physical labor, and a history of regular sports participation that can cause abnormal wear and tear of the knee joints.

The Hips

- Obesity and hip injury are important risk factors. Injury is more likely to create a problem in one hip.
- Among men, occupations that combine knee bending and heavy lifting can increase the risk of hip arthritis. Among women, working in a standing position may lead to more arthritis. European studies have shown a particularly high incidence of hip arthritis among farmers. Construction workers and firefighters also have a higher risk.

The Spine

- There are little data on the incidence of osteoarthritis of the spine, however the incidence may be much higher than anyplace else in the body. According to one study of a random sampling of 6,585 X rays of Dutch villagers, mild to severe arthritis in the neck and lower back were far and away the most common sites of joint degeneration in elderly people. The researchers from Erasmus University in Rotterdam commented that their data was comparable to ten other population surveys.

the risk factors

Many experts, such as David T. Felson, M.D., of Boston University's Arthritis Center, suggest an evolutionary explanation as to why the hands, feet, knees, hips, and spine are the joints most affected. The theory goes that from apes who walked using their upper extremities, we evolved into upright bipeds, putting the greatest stresses on the weight-bearing joints. Secondly, as we developed a pincer grip, the joints in our hands became vulnerable to degeneration.

According to archaeological evidence of human bone remains, joint wear and tear appears to have increased somewhat with the advent of the agricultural revolution (roughly ten thousand years ago). As people evolved into farmers, they began performing more laborious tasks requiring repeated motions of the same joints. As hunter-gatherers or small-scale agriculturists, they carried out a wider range of activities each day that promoted a healthier musculoskeletal system.

Arthritic deformities have been detected in the bones of early man and X rays of Egyptian mummies. Physicians in Greek and Roman times treated and described arthritis. At the time of the Romans, most people died by the age of twenty-five. And apparently 70 percent of those who lived longer than thirty experienced some form of arthritis.

Now, living into the eighties and nineties is not unusual. Such longevity gives us ample chance to develop the degenerative arthritis that typically has been many years in the making.

Experts don't know exactly why some people develop arthritis sooner, and others later, or why some don't experience symptoms even though X rays reveal a lot of degeneration. The only thing for sure is that we all get osteoarthritis sooner or later.

It would seem that such differences have many roots:

- the structural and biochemical weaknesses and strengths we inherit
- the influences of lifestyle
- individual tolerance for pain that prompts people to see their doctors

Just as there are risk factors for cardiovascular disease, there are also risk factors for osteoarthritis. And such risk factors are different for different joints. For instance, an injured football knee heightens the risk for osteoarthritis in that joint but not in the elbow. Some factors, as Felson points out, "may have purely local effects, whereas others have systemic effects."

Even when doctors take detailed medical histories and spend time with patients, it is hard to do more than suggest probable causes. But such information can provide important clues for heading off symptoms or stopping progression of the disease.

In today's harried medical world, and with the emphasis on disease care, physicians often don't have the time to help you figure out the cause of your problem or help you structure a prevention strategy. Finding a cause-oriented doctor is definitely in your best interest.

Robert E. Markison, M.D., a San Francisco hand surgeon and specialist in overuse disorders of the upper extremities, correctly points out that "people need guidance and a physician who can look and listen as opposed to simply prescribing an anti-inflammatory or other drug that leads to organ damage. Once the guidance is there, then it becomes a matter of 'self-rescue.'"

Following is a review of some of the main risk factors that can lead to osteoarthritis.

Wear and Tear

Osteoarthritis doesn't develop overnight. It takes time. Doing the same repeated motions many times a day for years, such as at work or in recreational pursuits, can create contact stress inside joints. This may result in microtrauma, subtle changes in joint biomechanics, and damage to cartilage. Certain occupational activities, for instance those that involve repetitive knee use and heavy lifting, raise the risk of arthritis in the knees and hips.

But we can also contribute to joint problems by some of the mindless ways we carry out daily activities, such as tilting our neck to cradle the phone while we talk, or slouching when watching television.

Acute Trauma (Injury)

Injury to a joint, even at an early age, creates a serious risk for osteoarthritis at the same site later in life.

Adolescents and young adults with traumatic injury to the knee joint, as well as persons with knee and hip injuries incurred during middle age, all face a much higher risk of arthritis. This revelation emerged from a study of three decades of medical data involving 1,321 former medical students at Johns Hopkins University.

The study, headed by Allan C. Gelber, M.D., Ph.D., was the first to analyze the relationship of joint injury in young people to the development of arthritis. Previous studies looked only at injuries in middle age or beyond. However, many athletic injuries occur in high school and college.

In sports and fitness, some activities carry with them a higher risk of joint damage. For instance, football, baseball pitching, volleyball, soccer, rugby, and martial arts such as karate may increase the risk because of direct and indirect impacts, injury to adjacent tissue (such as ligament tears), and repetitive twisting forces on the joints.

Female Gender

Arthritis is the leading chronic condition among women, and many more females suffer with it than men. At all ages of life, women have two to four times more osteoarthritis. When other types of arthritis and conditions that affect joints are factored in, the disproportion is even higher—as much as ten times higher. Women also experience higher rates of arthritis-related consequences. For those over forty-five, it is the leading cause of activity limitation. Moreover, researchers say that women are more likely than men to report pain, and to feel less able to deal with it.

Obese women are at an especially higher risk of knee osteoarthritis, whereas obese men have a marginally higher risk than nonobese men. The difference, according to experts, may be due partly to the fact that thin men have a more frequent history of knee injury that leads to osteoarthritis. At this time, the reason for the disproportionate prevalence among women is not clearly understood, nor have any convincing explanations been established.

Is there an estrogen connection? Since elderly women are more prone to osteoarthritis than elderly men, researchers have scoured statistical data to find a possible estrogen role. Estrogen has major influences on more than three hundred tissue systems throughout the body, including the bones, where it has a protective effect. In the years just before and during menopause, the estrogen level declines dramatically in a woman's body.

The research has focused on menopausal women who use estrogen replacement (ERT) prescriptions in comparison to nonusers. Results have been somewhat mixed, favoring a nonsignificant protective effect for ERT.

Standard ERT, in any case, involves unnatural, chemicalized pharmaceutical formulas that do not resemble a woman's own hormones. It would be interesting to see if natural estrogen replacement might have a greater protective effect against osteoarthritis after fifty. I wonder also if natural progesterone would help if it were added to the mix. Women generally start to make less progesterone in their early thirties, and the decline accelerates over the ensuing years. Progesterone helps create new bone cells.

Overweight and Obesity

Excess pounds mean excess mechanical stress for the weight-bearing joints of the body. And that is a clear invitation for osteoarthritis.

Unfortunately, overweight and obesity are increasing dramatically in the United States and contribute in a huge way to chronic health conditions, impaired quality of life, and death, according to recent population studies. Weight problems are strongly linked to an increased risk of diabetes, high blood pressure, cardiovascular disease, and osteoarthritis.

It may be hard to believe, but more than half of all American adults are considered overweight or obese—63 percent of men and 55 percent of women! The rise of obesity, from an estimated 14.5 percent of the population in 1976–80 to 22.5 percent in 1988–94, has taken place despite popular diets and efforts by physicians to keep weight down among their patients. The rise in weight involves all states, both sexes, across all age groups, races, and educational levels.

The continuing fattening of America figures to contribute in a big way to the predicted osteoarthritis epidemic. Excess body weight leads to osteoarthritis of both knees, and may increase arthritic risk in the hips and, according to some studies, even the hands.

Arthritis expert David Felson has commented that "increased joint stress accompanying obesity may explain the strong linkage between obesity and knee osteoarthritis risk, (but) it does not necessarily explain why obese people are at higher comparative risk of disease in the hand nor why obese women are at higher comparative risk of knee disease than obese men. Unfortunately, studies of metabolic factors linked to obesity have not provided an explanation for these findings." One suggestion in this area is that in obese individuals, excess fat tissue may produce abnormal levels of certain hormones or growth factors affecting cartilage or underlying bone in a way that promotes the risk of osteoarthritis.

Obesity in middle age is known to increase the risk of osteoarthritis of the knees in later life. What about obesity in younger years? Researchers have recently found that excess weight at a younger age—twenty to twenty-nine—is even more predictive of future arthritis!

And against this revelation is the alarming rise of childhood obesity in the United States and other industrialized countries. Among American children, estimates range from 11 to 25 percent. In China, the incidence is "out of control," according to one study. The problem is that very heavy children tend to be very heavy adults.

Just in case you aren't sure you are overweight, a simple formula in chapter 8—the chapter on eating right—can give you an instant verdict according to a standard called the body mass index.

Genetics

For more than a half-century, medical researchers have felt that osteoarthritis onset and progression involves some degree of genetic predisposition. But exactly how large an influence is still an issue of speculation. Timothy Spector, M.D., and F. M. Cicuttini, M.D., of Australia's Monash University, say the genetic influence may relate to a structural defect in collagen that makes a person more prone to early arthritis or alterations in cartilage or bone metabolism. Such a defect could also accentuate a risk factor like obesity.

Even though severe osteoarthritis may be common in your family, you aren't automatically pegged for a similar fate. I have seen many patients who came from parents with severe arthritis, but who did not develop chronic symptoms. They made many of the lifestyle recommendations I discuss later in this book and I believe this helped them delay or minimize joint problems.

Free-Radical Activity

Oxygen, as we all know, is essential to survival. It fuels the critical metabolic reactions in our body that generate energy for motion, sensation, and thought. This basic-to-life oxidative process, in which oxygen burns glucose molecules to create energy, is conducted in every cell. However, it creates dangerous by-products down at the cellular level—free radicals. They are unstable, highly reactive molecular combinations of oxygen and other atoms that "kidnap" electrons from surrounding atoms or molecules. Unless contained by the body's own natural antioxidants and repair mechanisms, free-radical activity can unleash a destructive blitz of oxidation that over time takes a heavy toll on healthy cells, tissues, and eventually bodily functions.

Free-radical activity is intimately involved in numerous ailments, such as cancer, vascular and heart disease, emphysema, adult-onset diabetes, ulcers, cataracts, Crohn's disease, senility, the very inflammatory rheumatoid arthritis, and osteoarthritis as well.

To get an idea of this destructive side to our precious oxygen, just consider how oxygen spoils food, turns butter rancid, and rusts metal. Lifestyle habits and the world we live in generate free-radical opportunities galore. Stress, smoking, alcohol, excess exposure to sunlight, excess exercise, chemical contaminants, pesticides, chemotherapy and pharmaceutical drugs, and processed, smoked, or barbecued foods—all increase free-radical production and create dangerous overloads in the body.

Moreover, our bodies seem to produce more free radicals as we get older, according to University of Nebraska's Denham Harman, M.D., Ph.D., originator of the free-radical theory of aging.

Free radicals attack DNA, enzymes, and proteins and disrupt normal cellular activities. They oxidize the fatty part of cell membranes, a process called lipid peroxidation. In the cells lining arterial walls, prolonged activity of this nature promotes hardening and thickening of the blood vessels and contributes to heart attacks and stroke. Free-radical activity unleashed by radiation from the sun can decrease skin suppleness and increase wrinkling.

There is also a positive side to free radicals: They are produced by the immune system as ammunition to destroy harmful microorganisms that enter the body, such as bacteria and viruses.

In recent years, researchers have conducted laboratory experiments with animal and human chondrocyte cells that demonstrate that free-radical oxidative damage occurs in osteoarthritis. Certain free radicals, for instance, degrade the proteoglycans and collagen produced by the chondrocytes. The free-radical activity is thought to contribute to the progression of osteoarthritis, rather than the initiation, and may be a consequence of tissue damage.

Nutrition

Research on nutrition and osteoarthritis is just beginning, and the early data suggest that good nutrition has a preventive role. The whole body, joints included, benefits from good nutrition. Moreover, certain supplements exert protective or therapeutic effects directly in the joints. In recent years, glucosamine and MSM (methylsufonylmethane) have captured a good deal of attention from patients, but there are other beneficial supplements you should also know about. I'll cover them in chapter 9.

Muscle Weakness

Muscles play a major role in the operation of our joints. Muscle activity and placement around joints provide mobility, stability, shock absorption, and control of movement. Weak muscles fatigue more readily and compromise the many protective mechanisms of the joints.

Researchers are starting to look at muscle weakness and dysfunction as risk factors for osteoarthritis. Among them is Michael Hurley, Ph.D., of King's College in London, who has theorized a scenario for how muscle weakness leads to osteoarthritis:

1. Weak muscles contribute to excessive joint movement and instability.
2. This creates jarring and irregular pressures on the joints, resulting in irritation of local nerve tissue, pain, and microtrauma of cartilage and bone tissue beneath the cartilage.
3. Stiffness occurs over time in the subcartilage bone tissue, which "becomes an anvil" on which cartilage is pounded, causing further damage.

"The joint can become embroiled in a circle of pathological events whereby even relatively minor joint damage can progress to severe joint degeneration," Hurley wrote in a 1999 article in the journal *Rheumatic Disease Clinics of North America.*

While this sequence of events is speculative, the idea of muscle weakness initiating joint damage and pain seems logical. Lack of exercise contributes to muscle weakness. Thus, for both arthritis prevention and therapy, exercise is an essential activity. Muscle weakness can also be caused by injury and disuse during convalescence.

One muscle where the connection has been clearly made is the quadriceps, the large muscle in the front of the thigh. Weakness here has been linked to knee arthritis in women.

Myths About Arthritis

STIFFNESS

Many people as they get older experience stiffness in the morning. Or, after sitting in a chair for a while, feel a little stiff when they arise.

"That means I've got arthritis, doesn't it, Doc?" patients will ask.

The reality: not necessarily.

Usually, these episodes of stiffness are brief. The stiffness disappears or diminishes substantially after you are up and moving around for a while.

Brief morning stiffness or stiffness that occurs with inactivity are commonly thought to be arthritis. More often than not, it is muscle stiffness, which comes with aging. Afterward you feel fine. That's not arthritis.

If you did a lot of gardening the day before and then wake up stiff, you have myositis—muscle inflammation. That's not arthritis either. You probably were using muscles you normally don't use.

You have arthritis if joint pain persists or occurs intermittently throughout the day.

THE WEATHER

Many people believe that a cold, damp climate can cause arthritis or make arthritis pain worse.

The reality: There is plenty of arthritis in warm climates. One study found that arthritic patients in mild San Diego had as much pain as patients in the colder clime of Boston. All the risk factors for osteoarthritis are present in the arctic and on the equator. Scientific research hasn't been able to prove a connection between bad weather and arthritis.

Arthritics tend to feel better in a warmer climate, which may also promote more activity. Physical activity is both a preventive and therapeutic factor for arthritis.

Soaking in a Jacuzzi, taking a hot shower, and applying moist hot packs to affected joints are always soothing.

ONLY MINOR ACHES AND PAINS

Television commercials give the impression that relief for "the minor aches and pains" of arthritis is just an aspirin or Tylenol away.

The reality: Over-the-counter medications are helpful in many cases, and may be all that a person needs. But a huge number of people suffer from much more severe pain requiring strong painkilling drugs.

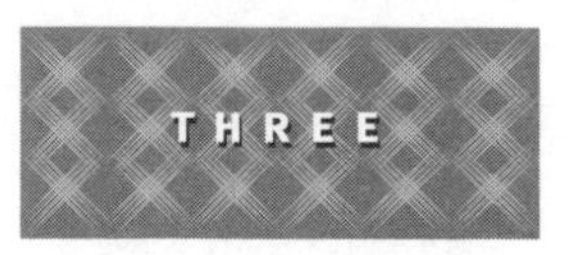

The High Price of Pain Relief

- "The pain is so bad that I don't want to get out of bed. I am even afraid of moving."
- "I hurt so much that I can't even play with my grandchildren. The pain has taken away a great source of joy in my life."
- "Because of the pain I am irritable all the time and grouchy with people I love."
- "I can't have intercourse because my back and knees are so painful."
- "The pain in my knee distracts me to the point where it is really interfering with my job performance."
- "The pain is so bad that it is hardly worth living anymore."
- "You are my last hope."

Over the years I have repeatedly heard these comments.

Can we physicians provide significant relief for such suffering? Many patients are lulled into a false sense of security regarding our ability to treat the pain. They think that medical science has all the answers—the magic pill or miracle surgery—and that the doctor will rescue them.

Some patients are so desperate for relief that they readily take the most powerful of painkillers and become addicted to them, with no concern about the side effects. Or they submit to any surgical procedure.

Cartilage doesn't have a nerve supply. The pain in osteoarthritis is thought to come from inflammation in the nerve-rich synovial lining of the joint, microfractures in the bone tissue just beneath the cartilage that often accompany arthritis, or pressure against nerve endings created by calcium spurs. Whatever the precise reason or reasons, the results can be excruciating. Most people with osteoarthritis seek medical attention because of the pain. That's why they come to see me—a pain specialist.

We indeed have powerful tools at our disposal today. But even the wonders of modern medicine have a sobering downside and a price to pay for pain relief.

medication

The parade of painkillers begins with aspirin for early pain, followed by the stronger medications, and then, for really severe conditions, the narcotic analgesics. While performing the humane mission of eliminating pain, these drugs are neither corrective nor preventive. And in order to be strong enough to do the job, they are often counterproductive to healing:

- They create well-documented toxicity in the body.
- They interfere with normal metabolic activities.
- They cause puzzling, misleading, or new symptoms that often mimic other diseases.
- They can interfere with a physician's treatment and distort laboratory readings.
- And they can even be deadly.

As a young physician treating arthritics back in the 1950s, I did what most other physicians did at the time: prescribe aspirin and moist heat applications. These are two standards of treatment that I still recommend. In those early days, we would also suggest purchasing topical analgesics such as BenGay for added relief. If these simpler approaches didn't work, patients didn't have many other options.

Sometime around the mid-1950s we started using phenylbutazone, a drug we welcomed as an exciting new answer to degenerative arthritis pain. I did some of the initial research with the drug for hip arthritis. It was quite effective, relieving about 90 percent of pain, much like today's new drugs. But soon we became aware of ugly side effects, including hemorrhaging under the skin.

I remember prescribing a standard dose for a female patient who had developed osteoarthritis at a young age because of obesity. She was in her early forties, five-foot-two, and 350 pounds, with bad pain in her back, knees, and ankles. She returned within a month in a shocking state. Large parts of her body were a deep purple color, the result of hemorrhaging capillaries. It took months for the discoloration to disappear.

The drug also had a toxic effect on the immune system's white blood cells, and we began to see patients developing leukemia-like symptoms and infections.

In the early 1960s, the U.S. Food and Drug Administration (FDA), the agency responsible for approval of medical drugs, started taking a hard stand because of the thalidomide scare. Thalidomide was a sedative widely used in Europe that was discovered to cause serious deformities of the fetus when used during pregnancy. As thalidomide horror stories spread, the emerging side effects of phenylbutazone prompted physicians to back off the new painkiller.

Then cortisone became available. This medication was the pharmaceutical version of cortisol, the anti-inflammatory steroid hormone produced in the adrenal glands. Here was the new answer to pain and inflammation, physicians were told.

We used pure cortisone in the beginning—hydrocortisone acetate.

But soon we started to see side effects when the drug was given orally: bleeding from the bowel, black stools, vomiting and nausea, ulcers, increased susceptibility to infections, as well as mental disturbances such as delusion and paranoia. We saw patients develop textural changes in the skin and a characteristic puffy, moonlike face. We found we could often overcome these problems by using smaller doses or reserving cortisone just for advanced cases.

Later, the intra-articular cortisone injection was developed, an effective method still widely used. It involves injecting cortisone into an affected joint to relieve pain and knock down inflammation. One injection often eliminates pain for a considerable length of time. Some patients need only one a year, while others need it more often. Physicians don't like using the injection more than a few times a year at the most. That's because multiple injections can accelerate cartilage degeneration. If a patient is quite elderly, more injections might be an acceptable trade-off. In any case, such usage should be monitored carefully.

NSAIDs—less pain but new problems

Pharmaceutical companies continually introduce new drugs. The next big wave brought us the nonsteroidal anti-inflammatories—NSAIDs (en-sayds), for short. The industry was seeking the same impact of cortisone but without the side effects. Indeed, the particular side effects associated with cortisone were eliminated, but a new and serious set of adverse reactions cropped up instead: stomach bleeding, ulcers, kidney damage, and hypertension.

Today, NSAIDs are among the most widely used medications for pain in the world. Typically, if you start to experience some joint pain today, you probably will try over-the-counter NSAIDs first. Among them are aspirin and products like Advil, Aleve, Motrin-IB, and Nuprin. Even these well-known products can cause problems when taken frequently or in higher doses than recommended.

NSAIDs block the action of an enzyme called cyclooxygenase. The enzyme produces hormonelike substances called prostaglandins that have central roles in pain and inflammation. NSAIDs also interfere with prostaglandins that protect the lining of the stomach. This allows gastric juices to damage the lining. Gastrointestinal disease is, in fact, regarded as the most common serious drug side effect in the United States.

A sophisticated 1999 British study published in the journal *Gut* revealed that NSAID formulations caused harmful changes in the digestive tract of nearly half of 312 patients using them for arthritis and other conditions. Twenty percent of these individuals showed inflammation akin to inflammatory bowel disease.

In the same year, an American study published in the journal *Clinical Therapeutics* reported significant gastrointestinal changes in 37 percent, and ulcers in 24 percent, of 1,826 arthritis patients taking NSAIDs. The incidence of ulcers was found to increase with age, duration of osteoarthritis, and medication use. The researchers said their evidence supports the contention that "safer treatment alternatives to conventional NSAIDs are required."

At a 1997 American Medical Association conference on pain, experts said that the overuse of many common prescription and over-the-counter NSAIDs was a "public health problem." The statistics certainly bear that out:

- A total of 50 to 80 percent of people admitted to hospitals with gastrointestinal bleeding are taking NSAIDs.
- Such patients have a 10 percent chance of dying.
- An estimated 13 million individuals take NSAIDs in the United States, the majority of whom have osteoarthritis. This usage sends about 107,000 patients to hospitals each year with gastrointestinal complications, according to "conservative calculations" from a major multimedical center study reported in the *American Journal of Med-*

icine in 1998. At least 16,500 deaths occur among arthritis patients alone who are taking NSAIDs. "The figure for all NSAID users would be overwhelming, yet the scope of the problem is generally underappreciated," wrote Gurkirpal Singh, M.D., of Stanford University.

- Evidence has appeared recently suggesting NSAIDs may also contribute to the development of congestive heart failure in elderly patients with a history of cardiovascular disease. This may be an "underrecognized public health problem," and "NSAIDs should be used with caution" among such patients, concluded a report by researchers at Australia's University of Newcastle that appeared in the *Annals of Internal Medicine*.

NSAIDs provide pain relief for as long as they are used, which, for obvious reasons, should not be long. The Arthritis Foundation says no longer than thirty days at a time.

Newer anti-inflammatory medications (COX-2 inhibitors) supposedly have fewer side effects. However, their cost is prohibitive—four dollars a pill. Monthly, that's a $300–$400 expense for a patient. The research claims these new NSAIDs will reduce by half the adverse reactions of their predecessors. If time proves this to be true, it would be a major and welcome reduction. But does that mean they will cause only (!!!) eight thousand deaths and fifty thousand or so hospital admissions a year? Is that acceptable?

Moreover, drugs usually appear safer when first introduced. Then, with more use over time, and patients requiring higher potencies to obtain results, a more disturbing picture of side effects tends to surface.

The manufacturers of the new generation of anti-inflammatories, such as Vioxx and Celebrex, spend millions of dollars in advertising their products to the public. You've probably seen them advertised on television in those corny commercials where symptomatic seniors are transformed into pain-free playmates for their grandchildren.

While recently watching *60 Minutes*, one of the most widely viewed programs on television, I counted five commercials pitching prescription drugs, including arthritis painkillers. After such shows I find patients asking for the drugs they have seen advertised. In other countries, advertising medical drugs on television and in the lay media is not permitted. But it's OK in the United States. Such advertising may be appropriate for aspirin, but not for strong prescription medication that needs to be evaluated for usage by a trained physician.

Another type of over-the-counter preparation is the familiar Tylenol, an acetaminophen compound. This product is loosely grouped into the NSAID category but does not inhibit prostaglandins or promote damage in the stomach. Acetaminophen helps relieve pain. It is less effective against inflammation, and some people, particularly heavy drinkers, may experience liver damage from high doses taken long term. On balance, Tylenol is a reasonably safe medication. If it works to control your arthritic pain, it is worth taking.

Many arthritic patients have difficulty falling sleeping, or are frequently woken up during the night, because of the pain. In a 1996 Gallup survey commissioned by the National Sleep Foundation, 60 percent of the respondents over age fifty experienced arthritic pain at night. All respondents over fifty with nighttime pain of any kind and who also had difficulty sleeping lost an average of nearly eleven nights of sleep in a typical month!

According to the poll, the vast majority of these individuals used some type of medication, either over-the-counter or prescription, to remedy their discomfort and sleeplessness. Their medication ranged from aspirin and Tylenol to strong narcotic prescriptions containing codeine. The original codeine medications used by physicians caused constipation. Improved versions—such as the current dihydrocodone—reduce the problem. There is, however, a risk of addiction, as well as a tolerance factor. That means the body gets accustomed to the medication and then you need more to generate the same painkilling effect. Vicodin is the best known brand in this group.

lessons from fifty years of prescribing painkillers

During my half-century in medical practice I have prescribed virtually every painkiller to come off the pharmaceutical assembly line. Initially, many of them were touted as "miracle drugs." Time and usage, however, revealed the overwhelming majority of them to be flawed.

Years ago, we were far less aware than today of the significance of drug side effects. Often the side effects were thought to be signs of the aging or disease process. Although there were many physicians who correctly voiced concern, it has only been within the last twenty years that the issue has been studied seriously and taken on major importance.

Adverse drug events, as side effects are called in medical parlance, are now thought to be much more common than previously believed. Medical drugs represent the fourth leading cause of death in U.S. hospitals, after heart disease, cancer, and stroke. The reliance on a pharmaceutical standard in medicine exacts a huge price. Estimates of the economic fallout from drug-related injury and death range from $30 to $130 billion annually.

When you stop to consider the repercussions, it is inappropriate to think of painkillers as long-term remedies. In the short term they may be generally safe for most people to deal with acute pain. But you are sacrificing some aspect of your health if you use them indefinitely. Moreover, such pain relief does not correlate to a healing process. Scientific studies suggest that some of these drugs may even damage cartilage.

It is also well known that medication impairs the absorption of nutrients such as vitamins and minerals. Cortisone, for instance, can interfere with vitamin B6. Aspirin and cortisone interfere with vitamin C, which is vital for the production of collagen, an important component of healthy cartilage.

A physician needs to weigh carefully the price of pain relief for osteoarthritis. The price may be much more than what you pay for a prescription. Arthritics have to take medication continually—for the long haul, frequently for the rest of their lives. But if the price shortens life or makes a patient sick, is it worth it?

In my busy pain practice, the evidence of side effects convinced me early on to look for safe and effective alternatives. My quest led me to natural remedies, the judicious use of exercise, acupuncture, self-administered physiotherapy techniques, and other methods I discovered around the world. When integrated into my practice, these options dramatically widened my treatment horizons and allowed me to regularly reduce or even eliminate reliance on strong medications.

You may wonder why most physicians generally do not prescribe or recommend natural remedies for pain. The basic reason is that medicine, as practiced in this country, is almost totally influenced by the pharmaceutical industry. Pharmaceutical companies research, develop, and patent unique formulas, and then market the drugs with huge budgets to physicians and the public. The medications are often based on natural substances found in the body or in plants, then modified with add-on molecules to make them unique. The new unique compounds are patented to legally protect the investment and future profits by deterring another company from copying the formula.

Pharmaceutical researchers are interested in "active ingredients." They will synthesize, for instance, the main painkilling substance in an herb but ignore other natural compounds in the plant that give it a built-in check-and-balance quality. When alien molecules are added in the pharmaceutical process, the result is often a powerful but problematic new medication. Reports of drug toxicity are frequently in the news.

Many patients who develop side effects are prescribed additional drugs to counteract the side effects. And when patients develop emotional problems such as anxiety and depression, as occurs in many cases of chronic disease, physicians then prescribe additional medications.

Drugs. Drugs. And more drugs. The more you take, the more you promote unhealthy reactions in the body. Polypharmacy—multiple prescriptions—is a dangerous and murky practice. Any drug, from an aspirin to a powerful painkiller, alters the body as well as the actions of other drugs being taken in ways we don't always understand.

When I went into practice, patients had one family doctor who kept track of them. Today, that's becoming less and less common. Many people are enrolled in HMOs. They don't have a single family physician to oversee their care. If they do, the doctor is usually dealing with an overload of patients.

Too often patients don't tell their doctors about other medications they are taking, and too often, doctors don't ask. A new physician may add another drug to the mix.

Polydoctors lead to polypharmacy.

You may take the COX-2 inhibitor and be painfree for a while. Then all of a sudden you develop a bellyache and go to the doctor. The doctor says you have irritable bowel or maybe a little anxiety causing some stomach upset. So he gives you an antianxiety medication. Now you are taking two drugs. But you don't feel well. You feel depressed. And nobody tells you that antianxiety medicine can create some depression. The doctor now gives you an antidepressant. Ad infinitum.

Unfortunately, these situations are fairly common. Patients fall into a medical net and have a hard time extracting themselves from a tangle of confounding side effects.

Yes, drugs provide important relief. But they carry toxic baggage with them. As Joseph Beasley, M.D., former dean of the School of Public Health at Tulane University, has pointed out, medications "are not selective, and the complexity of the human organism makes it difficult if not impossible to predict exactly what a substance will do when taken into the body. Unfortunately, drug companies (and many physicians they indoctrinate) tend to the simplistic view of drugs as 'magic bullets' and gear their research, advertising, and treatment efforts accordingly."

But as Beasley warned in his landmark book, *The Kellogg Report: The Impact of Nutrition, Lifestyle and the Environment on the Health of Americans* (Bard College Center, 1989), the magic bullets can often act like "hand grenades" and do considerable damage.

surgery

In today's age of surgical wizardry, total joint replacement has become a medical bestseller. Arthroplasties, as the surgical procedures are formally called, have risen steadily since replacement techniques were first introduced in the 1970s. According to the American Academy of Orthopedic Surgeons, more than 700,000 upper and lower extremity arthroplasties are now performed annually, most of them involving knees and hips.

Nowadays, surgeons can replace your arthritic finger, hand, wrist, elbow, shoulder, hip, knee, ankle, foot, and toe joint with a new plastic or metallic prosthetic.

Many people see this as a quick fix. But it's not quick and it's not always a fix.

First of all, recovery from surgery and intensive physical therapy afterward can last for months. And the rosy vision of pain relief and restored joint function after rehabilitation does not always materialize. While 60 to 65 percent of patients have successful outcomes, the rest experience no improvement or their situation is even worse.

In the early days of arthroplasties, replacements lasted perhaps five to seven years. Today, you get more mileage but no lifetime warranty with your new joint. If you have a hip replacement at age fifty, don't expect it to be working when you are seventy-five or eighty. You will probably need a replacement of the replacement. Joints wear out after ten or fifteen years, and the outcome of a second (or third) procedure is almost never as good as the first. In addition, surgery risks are greater with age.

I have also seen many people with problems afterward. Not infrequently, the legs are uneven, and people are left walking almost as if one foot is on the curb and the other on the street. The imbalance creates muscular and joint stresses elsewhere, leading to discomfort and pain. I would guess that one out of two of my patients developed back pain after knee or hip replacement.

Don't misunderstand me. This is a remarkable advancement for rehabilitating people in pain. I am not against the procedure. Many of my patients have benefited from it and I certainly recommend replacement when there are clear medical indications for it.

But it is no panacea.

There are many cases when replacement surgery is chosen even when there are other, less invasive, options. Recently, a thirty-five-year-old patient chose to have hip surgery—unwarranted in my opinion—only because she had some moderate degenerative changes and what she considered to be unbearable pain. I told her to consider different remedies to slow down the degeneration and delay the need for surgery, but she simply wanted to get it over with.

In addition to replacements, there is a popular surgical procedure known as arthroscopy. In these operations, orthopedic surgeons go into the joint area and, using microscopic techniques, clean up debris such as damaged cartilage, ligaments, and tendons. They are often very successful.

Physicians also use this technique to remove calcium deposits that are causing considerable joint pain. Unfortunately, though, the deposits return at some later date. This condition is somewhat similar to what happens with coronary artery surgery. If a patient doesn't change diet or lifestyle, the arteries will block up again within two to five years.

Removing calcium surgically provides temporary relief. The underlying pathology—the reason that the calcium is there in the first place—has not been addressed.

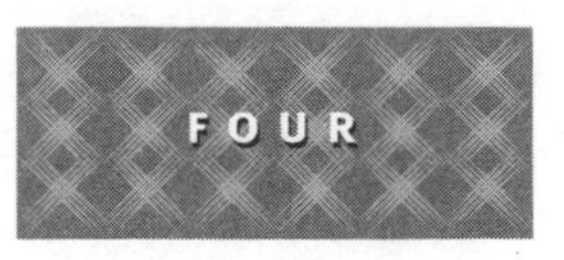

The Pandora's Box of Compounded Misery

As a young doctor I used to make house calls, including many at one particular trailer park populated by retirees. I can still remember seeing those elderly people sitting on the porches of their homes and just kind of rusting away.

I noticed that the arthritics among them had become increasingly inactive. It was more comfortable for them to just sit still. Obviously, you don't want to move a joint as much if it hurts you. The result is that you do less so that you have less pain. Back in those days, doctors told their patients to rest and not push themselves if they had painful arthritis. But the more those people sat around, the worse their arthritis would get.

Then and now, osteoarthritis symptoms commonly sideline people from life. The symptoms open a Pandora's box of misery, vicious cycles, and health-sapping consequences.

I have already discussed the issue of medication side effects and the complications of replacement surgery. But there are plenty of other nasty problems beyond pain associated with arthritis. They include:

- inactivity
- the loss of physical conditioning, a major risk factor for weight gain and life-threatening diseases
- reduced range of motion in affected joints

- physical disability, where simple basic tasks become harder to perform
- growing reliance on others
- a sense of being handicapped and, with it, a loss of emotional well-being
- reluctance to get out and socialize
- for patients of working age, lost workdays and productivity

Arthritis, with a domino effect of consequences, can cast a huge shadow on the burden of illness. These consequences speak volumes for the importance of prevention.

the inactivity connection

Among adults, arthritis is the leading cause of activity limitation. About 12 percent of people over the age of sixty-five are affected.

Within our body, movement is critical for joint and overall health. Movement promotes the good flow of blood and the delivery of nutrients. It stimulates lymph flow and with it the removal of waste products. A normal degree of "loading," the term for the mechanical forces applied to the joints during movement, stimulates the chondrocytes (the cartilage cells) to form resilient cartilage tissue.

Immobility does the opposite. It slows down cartilage production, nutrient delivery, and waste product removal. Disuse makes cartilage more susceptible to injury and atrophy. If disuse is prolonged, cartilage integrity is jeopardized and normal joint function reduced as the joint capsule becomes overrun by fibrous tissue.

Both inside and outside the joint, the domino effect of inactivity is horrendous. It creates decreased physical fitness, immobility, impaired function, reduced muscle efficiency, loss of stability and range of motion in the joints, disability, obesity, the increased risk of developing other conditions, and increased use of medication. And all these, in turn, lead to more inactivity and a worsening of the underlying arthritic condition.

A 1996 article in the medical journal *Rheumatic Disease Clinics of North America* summed up the situation thus: "For the person with arthritis, the consequences of prolonged inactivity add measurably, and unnecessarily, to disease-related impairments, functional limitation, and disability. Inadequate levels of regular physical activity also increase the risk of cardiovascular disease, hypertension, diabetes and obesity."

And a higher risk for premature death, I should add.

the cardiovascular connection

The Surgeon General's Report on Physical Activity and Health in 1996 pointed out that inactivity is a primary risk factor for cardiovascular disease, the country's top disease killer. In a search of the medical literature I found more than a thousand scientific papers dealing with physical inactivity as a primary cause for cardiac and/or vascular disease.

The findings include evidence that inactivity secondary to arthritic symptoms sets up a higher risk for cardiovascular disease. For instance, at the Columbia University College of Physicians and Surgeons, forty-six patients with osteoarthritis of the hip and/or knee were compared to a matched group of nonarthritics. The researchers wanted to know if risk factors are higher for coronary heart disease among arthritis patients. They concluded that indeed patients with moderately severe or end-stage lower-extremity arthritis may be at advanced risk because of unfavorable risk factors. Such patients are severely deconditioned from a cardiovascular standpoint.

When you are inactive, whether it is from arthritis or simply leading a sedentary lifestyle, the circulation decreases. Cardiac output drops off. The heart loses conditioning and cannot pump out the necessary amount of blood, and the oxygen and nutrients it carries, to reach peripheral or end tissues.

A problem with blood flow opens the door to many problems. When cells don't get their share of essential needs, they function poorly, or they die. Stroke, for instance, is a result of not enough blood reaching the brain. Physical inactivity is one of several well-established risk factors for stroke.

the cancer connection

As the founding president of the American Medical Athletic Association, I began encouraging physicians more than thirty years ago to become more involved in exercise for their own good health.

After about ten years, I began suspecting a connection between inactivity and cancer, and particularly bowel cancer. I noted that the doctors who were the most active seemed to have a lesser incidence of cancer than my patients of the same age who had similar intense professional lives and stress levels.

Cancer is an anaerobic disease. That means it flourishes in tissues where the oxygen supply is diminished. Seventy years ago, the great German biochemist Otto Warburg was awarded a Nobel Prize for his research showing that lack of oxygen in normal body cells is a prime cause of cancer.

Exercise is obviously one way to move oxygen through the thousands of miles of blood vessels to the tissues. Inactivity, on the other hand, promotes stagnation and pooling of blood, and poor distribution of oxygen throughout the system.

In recent years, scientific evidence has pointed to a connection between inactivity and a heightened risk of certain cancers, such as colon, breast, lung, and prostate cancer. A recent Harvard University study, for instance, indicated that people with the highest level of physical activity had half the incidence of colon cancer as those who exercised the least. The researchers recommended more attention be given to exercise as a means of preventing the disease.

After reviewing 4,500 relevant scientific studies, a panel of experts assembled in 1997 by the American Institute for Cancer Research concluded that a "general association" exists between inactivity and overall cancer risk. According to the panel, there is "convincing evidence that physical activity decreases the risk of colon cancer and possibly breast and lung cancer. Conversely, obesity, often linked to inactivity, increases the risk of cancer of the kidney, endometrium, breast, bladder, colon and rectum."

the "use it or lose it" connection

Muscle is meant to be maintained in good condition through regular exercise. People who do so deteriorate physically at about a 5 percent rate per decade after "peaking" at about the age of twenty. People who do not exercise deteriorate much more rapidly.

An inactive life, as a by-product of arthritis, can result in a rapid shrinkage of muscles and a loss of response to normal everyday challenges. This debility is called disuse atrophy of the muscles.

The old admonition to "use it or lose it" surely applies to the human musculoskeletal system. Just thirty days of disuse can result in deterioration requiring as long as two years to restore. Muscle weakness, as I discussed in chapter 2, is now being regarded as an important risk factor. Thus, it is both a risk factor and a consequence, part of the vicious cycle.

the disability connection

The impact of osteoarthritis on physical disability is well documented. In particular, older women appear to be hardest hit. They have more arthritis and more disability than their male counterparts, experts say.

The following studies shed light on the extent to which lives are affected.

A Canadian statistical study of more than 130,000 people found that arthritis-associated disability is almost twice that of circulatory disorders that include heart disease and stroke. As reported in a 1995 issue of *Arthritis Care and Research,* arthritic patients were affected in this way:

- 25 percent could not leave their residence or could leave only with help.
- 45 percent had at least some level of physical dependence.
- 18 percent were not participating in social activities.
- 51 percent of those under age sixty-five were not in the labor force.
- 76 percent never went to events such as sports or movies.
- 42 percent had out-of-pocket expenses because of disability.

In a 1994 article in the *Journal of the American Geriatrics Society,* researchers surveyed a group of 9,700 ambulatory American women with arthritis living at home who were sixty-five or older. The women, questioned at different clinical centers, were asked if they had "any difficulty" performing six physical activities fundamental to daily living. The six activities were: (1) walking two to three blocks on level ground; (2) climbing up ten steps without stopping; (3) walking down ten steps; (4) preparing meals; (5) doing heavy housework; and (6) shopping for groceries or clothes.

The researchers, headed by Kristine E. Ensrud, M.D., of the Minneapolis Veterans Administration Medical Center, determined that osteoarthritis was the second leading cause for interference with the ability to carry out such tasks. A woman with arthritis, back pain, stroke, parkinsonism, hip or spine fracture was two to three times more likely to report impaired function than a woman without any of these conditions, she reported.

Barbara Downe-Wamboldt, R.N., of Dalhousie University in Nova

Scotia, visited ninety female arthritis patients in their homes to learn just how debilitating arthritis can be. The women she interviewed averaged 12.6 years since diagnosis. Her findings, reported in *Health Care for Women International,* concluded that osteoarthritis was extremely limiting in all respects for these women.

"A plan to visit at a friend's house, attend a community activity, or simply do the laundry was often abandoned because of the inability to get in and out of an automobile or to negotiate a few stairs," she wrote. "Routine tasks such as meeting self-care needs, housecleaning, and cooking were often problematic owing to pain and joint stiffness. Social activities with friends and family were affected and a diminished sense of independence was reported. As a result of living with osteoarthritis and the associated loss of function, these women had fewer choices in life, including work and leisure."

One more sobering thought: Studies indicate that arthritis-related disability and homeboundedness increase the risk for nursing home use. And nursing home care, as researchers from Northwestern University noted recently, "currently costs $35,000 per person per year and is financed out-of-pocket until the point of poverty, at which time care is reimbursed by Medicaid."

obesity

Here is a truly vicious cycle.

Excess weight promotes arthritic degeneration of the weight-bearing joints.

Arthritis leads to impaired function and reduced physical activity.

This, in turn, creates a higher risk for putting on more weight and developing cardiovascular disease and diabetes.

If you already have osteoarthritis of the knee, the additional weight will further exacerbate it.

stress

We are mind/body creatures and so the pain and impaired function of arthritis often leads to chronic stress, sleep disorders, anxiety, depression, and, as the disease progresses, to a growing perception of poor health.

On a biochemical level, chronic physical or emotional stress stimulates the adrenal glands to release the steroid hormone cortisol. Research has shown that excess cortisol, produced day after day as a result of chronic, unrelenting stress, damages and kills brain cells in the hippocampus by the billions. The hippocampus is an area of the brain related to learning and short-term memory. Such toxic overexposure is regarded as a contributor to memory loss and Alzheimer's disease.

Paul J. Rosch, M.D., president of the American Institute of Stress, and clinical professor of medicine and psychiatry at New York Medical College, says there is no question that a chronic high tide of cortisol contributes to an acceleration of the aging process and a host of stress-related disorders.

Rosch points out that there are a host of intricate interrelationships between stress and arthritis. "Some are so inextricably intertwined, that like the chicken and the egg, it's difficult to determine which came first," he says. "There is little doubt that arthritis can be severely stressful, because of disability, deformity, lowered self-esteem, and particularly pain. In turn, chronic stress can make individuals much more sensitive to pain, causing additional stress that intensifies the pain. A common example of this is seen in some patients with low back pain due to an arthritic spur on the spine, causing muscle spasm and nerve root pressure pain. Stress-induced muscle tension further increases this pressure, making the pain more severe, which in turn leads to more stress and greater discomfort and lack of mobility. The ability to relieve pain and/or to reduce stress, can relax tense muscles, breaking up this vicious and self-perpetuating cycle."

depression and anxiety

A significant minority of arthritic patients develops depression or anxiety and the additional disability and suffering they produce. Experts say this occurs in many serious chronic ailments. In the case of arthritis, it stems from the pain, increased physical limitation, fear of being immobile, and dread that the body is caught in an aging downslide to death.

Such stress-related complaints of arthritis patients commonly lead to overuse and dependency on drugs that have serious side effects and further reduce health.

Take the example of tranquilizers. For people over sixty-five, they are dangerous. They lead to further immobilization, reduction of oxygen uptake in the brain, and interference with basic processes of life and metabolism. Anxiety and sleeping medications increase the risk of disability, falls, and hip fractures. Yet the elderly commonly take these drugs.

Here, again, we have the dangerous practice of polypharmacy, taking multiple drugs. You start with arthritis medication and pile on more drugs for the collateral problems the disease produces.

PART II

ten steps for preventing arthritis

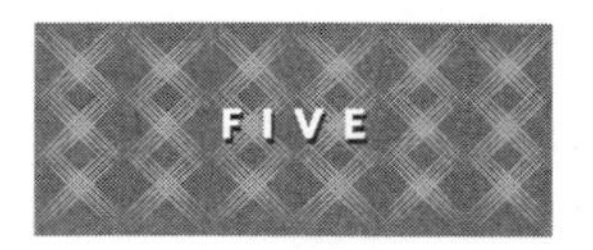

Stop the Strains from Becoming Pains*

Great oaks from small acorns grow, they say. And so, too, big pains from small strains grow.

That's my observation from decades of treating patients and observing how minor aches and strains from daily activity often develop over time into major musculoskeletal or arthritic pain.

Repetitive strain injuries (RSIs) have become a focus of medical attention in the workplace. They affect many people who perform the same repetitive motions day after day, year after year . . . motions such as gripping, twisting, bending, lifting, reaching, cutting, and keying. The National Institute of Occupational Safety and Health (NIOSH) says RSIs have increased dramatically in recent years because of automation and job specialization where a given job may involve only a few manipulations performed thousands of times per workday.

In completely different industries and jobs ranging from clerical and computer work to hard, physical labor, employees develop identical disorders because of the similar and repetitive ways they use their bodies. Unlike a sudden accident, these overuse conditions develop slowly and cause minute trauma to muscles, tendons, joints, and nerves. Over time, the damage builds up into severe pain, numbness, inflammation, restriction of joint movement, loss of strength and manual dexterity, and, if left untreated, lasting disability.

---

* See also chapter 12: Protect Your Hands

According to the U.S. Bureau of Labor Statistics, RSIs account for about 60 percent—and rank first—among all work-caused physical illnesses. The hazards and long-term consequences of RSIs are of particular concern to women. According to Bureau of Labor statistics, female workers account for nearly two-thirds of all work-related repetitive strain injuries even though women constitute only 45 percent of total employees.

Deborah Quilter, author of *The Repetitive Strain Injury Recovery Book* (Walker & Company, 1998), suggests that the higher risk to women is due to smaller and weaker muscles, hormonal changes in pregnancy and menopause, and work that frequently requires repetitive movements of the hands and arms, such as that of data entry operators, telephone operators, and cashiers. In addition, she says, women today are involved in more physically challenging jobs that previously were almost exclusively done by men.

In general, arms and shoulders may suffer because of fatiguing positions in which the arms are extended forward or upward. Examples are an auto mechanic working regularly beneath a hoisted car, or a supermarket cashier repeatedly and rapidly pulling merchandise over the scanner that reads the product bar code.

Long-term wear and tear on backs contributes in a big way to chronic pain, reduced mobility, sick leave, and early disability. Potentially harmful activities include bending, twisting, pushing, pulling, lifting, and lowering. Examples: an employee stacking products or a nurse lifting patients.

Manual tasks involving highly repetitive actions, or necessitating wrist bending or other stressful wrist postures, the use of vibrating tools and small hand tools, or long hours at the computer are notorious contributors to injuries of the hands, wrist, neck, forearm, and elbows.

Unfortunately, there is no way to predict who does and who doesn't develop an RSI, the experts say. Individuals respond differently to similar risk factors. Some people are more susceptible because of an existing health problem or physical characteristics that become aggravated by work activity.

In recent years, the dramatic rise in carpal tunnel syndrome and other disorders has focused much attention on ergonomics, a science that studies the way people can be affected by occupational tasks and conditions. Ergonomics is dedicated to the concept of fitting the work to the worker, so that the demands and conditions of the job do not exceed or strain an employee's capabilities.

Along with these developments, researchers have found that some occupational activities increase the risk of developing osteoarthritis and accelerate the progression of the disease if it is already present. Of course, keep in mind that work is just one part of life. There are other risk factors involved, and activities outside of work could have an even greater impact.

Here is what's known to date:

- Jobs involving repetitive heavy lifting, kneeling, and squatting significantly increase the risk of arthritis in the knee.
- Physical strain and standing on the job have also been related to an increased risk of arthritis in the hip.
- Farmers appear to have a higher risk for hip osteoarthritis.
- Abuse of joints by repetitive impacts can lead to progressive degeneration of cartilage.
- Normal use of abnormal joints, that is joints with irregular cartilage surfaces, misalignments, instability, or disturbed muscle nerve supply, may also increase the risk. "Some people may be born with defective cartilage or with slight defects in the way joints fit together," says the Arthritis Foundation. "As a person ages, these defects may cause early cartilage breakdown in the joint."
- Many athletes, as we will see in a later chapter, are at higher risk, but so too are many performers from the world of music and dance because of their long hours of practice and repeated motions. A new field of performing arts medicine has emerged in recent years to

study the musculoskeletal risks of performers. Researchers have found a statistically higher incidence of knee, ankle, and foot arthritis, including premature degeneration, among longtime or retired dancers than among nondancers. The investigators relate the prevalence to repetitive microtrauma. For musicians, many instruments can increase the risk of osteoarthritis in the hands. In pianists, for instance, the right hand has been reported to show early signs of degeneration.

how's your static level?

Forget your radio or cellular reception. I'm talking about your joints. Experts point to static muscular effort as a potential cause of joint problems. Static muscular work involves carrying the trunk, head, or limbs in unnatural, constrained postures for long periods of time.

According to Etienne Grandjean, of the Swiss Federal Institute of Technology, such static activities include bending the back either forward or sideways, holding objects in the arms, actions requiring the arms to be held out horizontally, putting weight on one leg while the other works a pedal, standing in one place for long periods, pushing and pulling heavy objects, and tilting the head strongly forward or backward.

In his book *Fitting the Task to the Man* (Taylor & Francis, 1988), Grandjean notes that some activities can be partly static and partly dynamic, such as computer work (see chapter 12 for more about computers).

"Shoulders and arms do mainly static work when holding the hands in the typing position, while the fingers perform mainly dynamic work when operating the keys," he points out. "Since static effort is much more strenuous than dynamic work, the static component of combined effort assumes greater importance. There is a static component in almost every form of physical work. Even moderate static work might produce troublesome localized fatigue in the muscles involved, which can build up to intolerable pain. If the static load is repeated daily over a long period, more or less permanent aches will appear in the limbs and may involve not only the muscles but also the joints, tendons and other tissues."

Grandjean states that static loads are associated with a higher risk of arthritis of the joints, and symptoms of degeneration, due to mechanical stress.

seek medical attention at first sign of problem . . . or even before

Prevention and symptom-reduction strategies include redesigning or customizing tools of the trade, modifying layouts of work stations, and special exercises and yoga postures (see chapter 11).

Even if you have undergone treatment for pain due to a structural stress, you may find yourself back in trouble if you don't change techniques and work habits that caused the problem in the first place. Recovery depends on how severe your case is, and how soon RSIs are properly diagnosed and treated. If you catch the problem early, your chances for complete recovery are better. If you wait too long, you may get relief of some symptoms but not regain full function.

As a member of the California Society of Industrial Medicine and Surgery, I have treated many musculoskeletal problems like this. I feel strongly that taking protective measures early on can help prevent microtrauma and repetitive injuries, and more serious problems later on. At the first sign of symptoms, be sure to see a competent physician immediately.

"You need a thorough diagnosis and a total health history from your doctor, to include anything from diabetes to thyroid disease to pregnancy, previous broken bones and injuries," says RSI expert Deborah Quilter. "All of these things—and your job demands—need to be evaluated by a physician who is competent to diagnose and treat RSI. You can't go by specialties, you have to go by the individual doctor's knowledge and expertise."

To find a good doctor, she suggests asking other people with RSIs for a referral. She also suggests contacting the Association of Occupational and Environmental Clinics in Washington, D.C. (phone: 202-347-4976). This organization can refer you to doctors knowledgeable about RSI or to support groups in your area.

In addition, there is a section on choosing doctors on Quilter's website, *www.rsihelp.com,* as well as other important information if you think you have an RSI.

People need to carefully read about treatments and methods, such as splinting, cortisone injections, and NSAIDs before they agree to them, she says, and adds: "Careful medical consumers need to know about the potential side effects of these methods. They are not usually done by the doctors who I believe to be on the leading edge of RSI rehabilitation. Many RSI patients go from doctor to doctor before they finally find the right person. Meanwhile they are getting worse."

One additional preventive point I'd like to recommend is an evaluation by an orthopedist, chiropractor, or podiatrist to determine any musculoskeletal abnormalities in the body. If you suspect a problem, don't wait for it to get worse. Abnormalities, over time, can exert harmful pressures on joints and promote arthritis. An evaluation, and corrective treatment, if necessary, could prevent a major problem in the future.

are you increasing your risk mindlessly?

Back in the mid-1950s, a female patient came to my office and complained of neck pain. She was about thirty and had had the pain for about five years. While interviewing her and taking down her medical history, I learned she was a secretary and spent a considerable amount of time on the phone with her head tilted to the side, bracing the receiver against her shoulder. A simple manual manipulation solved her pain problem and probably headed off degenerative arthritis down the line.

Her case alerted me to the importance of structural stresses. I began questioning patients about activities that might set them up for chronic pain and musculoskeletal problems.

I started analyzing even how people sat. I remember one young business executive who sat for hours every day in a poor-quality chair. He came in complaining of a chronic backache. It turned out that his chair didn't provide enough curvature for the back. I told him to take the telephone yellow pages and put the book on the floor under his feet. That, and a better chair, helped ease his back.

The yellow pages "cure" has helped hundreds of my patients over the years. This simple method protects the natural curve of the small of the back, preventing muscle and tendon pull on the vertebral joints. It is these forces that promote cartilage wear, disturbance in blood flow, and the formation of calcium in joints under tension.

These cases demonstrate how many of the most simple and mindless activities in our lives can contribute to years of chronic aches and muscular stresses. These, in turn, as I would tell my patients, are setting you up for decreased blood flow, increased muscle spasm, and compression of the joints. In other words, a fertile field for osteoarthritis.

As you read this book you may get the feeling that everything you do can lead to osteoarthritis. The truth is that if you repeat something enough it probably will cause wear and tear to some degree at some point. That's life.

Through X rays taken over time, it became quite clear to me how patient complaints of chronic aches and muscular stresses were often the forerunner for osteoarthritis. The stresses and strains represent microtrauma to the joints and surrounding tissue. Over the years they add up and one day you have osteoarthritis with pain.

Here are some daily—and potentially risky—actions and situations worth thinking about:

• Reading in Bed

I hope you are not reading this book in bed!

One largely unsuspected but leading cause of headaches is reading in bed. Kids do it. We all do it. We lie on our backs with a pillow propped under our head. The problem is that the head is bent forward at too sharp an angle. This unnatural position strains the muscles attached to the back of the skull and initiates a painful cycle of muscular tension, neckaches, and headaches. Over a long period of time, it can contribute to degenerative changes in the neck vertebrae, resulting in arthritic pain.

Reading while lying on your stomach, propped up on your elbows, also leads to marked neck and back strain as well as stress in the shoulder areas. I know from experience. This is the way I used to read years ago when I was a young man. And I do recall becoming achy on many occasions before I got smart.

If you insist on reading in bed, prop yourself up against a comfortable stack of pillows between you and the headboard or wall. Place a pillow under your knees. The pillow is important. Without one, your legs are resting flat on the bed straight out in front of you, putting stress on your lower back muscles.

• Lift Right or Pay the Price

Lower back pain has probably been the most common complaint among my patients. The most frequent cause is improper lifting.

You can stay out of trouble if you remember to use *all of you* when lifting. That means using your arms, body, and legs.

Most people tend to bend down and lift with their arms alone. This strains the lower back muscles and vertebral joints, often leading quickly to muscular aches. Keep that up and you will contribute to the eventual development of degenerative spinal arthritis and chronic pain. I have observed this progressive scenario in thousands of patients.

A typical case involved a forty-year-old warehouseman who lifted and carried boxes of merchandise at one of the large retail electronic stores near my office. He first came to see me complaining of an aching back that developed regularly at the end of his workday. X rays showed early signs of degeneration in the lower spine. I recommended a protective lumbar belt and instructed him on some protective lifting techniques.

About five years later, he returned, complaining this time of constant pain in his lower back. He woke up with it in the morning and it grew worse during the day. X rays now showed marked degeneration. Even though he had more support from the belt, and was quite careful in how he lifted boxes, microtrauma to the lower spine over the years had taken its toll.

It is not the weight of the object that does the damage. It is the way you lift. No matter how light an object appears to be, always bend at the knees, gently lower yourself into a squat position, and then lift with your entire body.

An initial injury is often brought on by rotating the trunk to lift something. That means instead of facing the object to be picked up, you pick it up by bending down and twisting to the left or right. Center yourself first so the object is directly in front of you. This enables you best to handle the weight in a balanced fashion. Otherwise, the spine receives an unequal force, the muscles on one or the other side of the lower back bear more weight, and you create structural stress that can lead to ligament and muscle injury, and subsequent pain.

• Overhead Lifting

I have treated many patients with osteoarthritis in the neck as a result of jobs in which they reach overhead and pull objects down. Obviously, a warehouseman would be an example. But I have treated many secretaries who have developed neck pain simply from having to reach up to shelves and pull down reference books frequently throughout their workday. If they have had pain for some time, their X rays or MRIs usually show evidence of degeneration in the cervical spine.

Neck pain is the third most common chronic pain problem, after lower back pain and headaches. As we get older, even sudden movements of the neck can damage ligaments, muscles, and bone and promote the development of chronic pain.

The simple motion of looking upward can be risky. I usually advise patients past age forty to exercise care when looking upward. Tasks such as changing a lightbulb or getting something off a high shelf should be performed while using a small step stool or ladder. Keep the head in as neutral a position as possible.

In extending the neck, such as in an upward gaze, older persons may have a tendency to get very dizzy. This can result in a fall, which might fracture a hip or other part of the body.

• "Telephonitis"

Depending on how you use your telephone, you may be paying more than you think for your calls. If you are not careful, your time on the phone can literally become a pain-in-the-neck. I have repeatedly treated patients for neck pain who habitually tilt their head to one side or the other to hold the telephone receiver against the shoulder while doing other things with their hands.

I have noticed this problem more with women than men. The pain will typically start around age thirty or thirty-five, the result of years of using a telephone in this manner. Many female patients have told me that they often file or polish their fingernails while on the phone.

If you need free hands while you talk, use a headset or speakerphone. Many contemporary phones are equipped with these features. Why torture your neck unnecessarily?

I would also advise parents to bring this up with their teenage children, who often spend hours on the phone talking to friends. If they hold the phone improperly, I can assure you they are on their way to developing chronic inflammatory changes in the neck. I have seen many men and women in their early twenties who have already developed arthritic changes or calcific deposits in the neck because of their telephone habits.

• "TVitis"

Do you spend a lot of time watching TV? If you do, and your TV posture is bad, you may be setting the stage for osteoarthritis.

Looking down, with your head bent, at the monitor for an hour or two a day will create eyestrain, neck tension, headaches, and the risk of degenerative arthritis in the neck. When you watch television, keep the monitor directly in your normal line of vision, or even slightly above. Don't watch while perched on a sofa or chair with the monitor on the floor.

I have treated many people in their twenties, and even younger, who were involved in vehicular accidents and was frequently shocked to find X ray evidence of arthritic changes in the neck. When I questioned them about their lifestyle, I was able to attribute some cases of degeneration to school sports injuries, such as in football. But most of the time there were no such injuries. Further questioning often revealed addicts who spend hours in front of a TV set in an improper position that creates chronic neck strain.

Many physicians have told me of finding similar X ray evidence of early arthritic changes in the necks of young patients being treated after accidents.

There is another problem involved here. We are rightly concerned about the amount of television our children watch because of the violence in programming as well as the sedentary behavior it encourages. We never think of television, however, in terms of osteoarthritis. But watching TV for many hours can be a double-barreled risk:

1. Strain on the back and neck produced by bad viewing posture.
2. The combination of snacking and inactivity produces fat kids. Research tells us that one in four children in the United States is obese, and obese children are more likely to develop into obese adults. Obesity raises the risk of osteoarthritis, as well as heart disease, diabetes, and other health problems.

sitting pretty

Humans were designed to be on the move and not sitting for as long as most of us do. But if we are going to sit for long we should be sure to give our bodies the best possible chair, whether we are working or driving.

Office chairs are improving, but they still contribute to many cases of backache among office workers. Chairs often have little more than a cushioned pad for midback support. That is not enough. You need a chair that can be adjusted to individual height, and the unique contour and curve of the lower back.

If you spend a lot of hours sitting, and can afford it, I recommend the Rolls-Royce of chairs—the award-winning Aeron chair, made by Herman Miller, Inc., of Zeeland, Michigan (phone: 888-443-4357; or on the Internet at *www.hermanmiller.com*). The Aeron has multiple adjustment features such as tilt, seat height, and movable armrests. Tilting back, for instance, allows you to avoid prolonged sitting in a single static position that reduces the natural pumping action of muscles to deliver nutrients to the intervertebral discs. Armrests and a reclining position help take a significant amount of upper-body weight load off the spine.

There are many other good chairs that offer adjustable features to eliminate or reduce strain and fatigue in the body. You can find them at specialty stores such as Relax the Back (*www.relaxtheback.com*).

Most people think of desk work as nontraumatic, yet I have treated many secretaries and office workers over the years who, as a result of sitting at a desk, developed chronic back and neck stresses that led to osteoarthritis.

If the company you work for won't seat you as comfortably as you would like, my advice is to buy a portable, folding orthopedic seat that is form-fitting and provides good total support for your back. Such seats are obtainable at orthopedic supply shops and can be shaped to your proper fit by store personnel.

These seats can also be used to increase neck and back comfort for less-than-perfect seats, including airline, theater, restaurant, and ballpark seats. I often see people carrying their folded orthopedic seats under their arms to places where poor seating might otherwise create strain or pain.

When seated for a prolonged period, never rest your feet flat on the floor. This transmits stress to the lower back. Instead, place something like the yellow pages under your feet. This elevates your knees and reduces stress. Tension on the lower back will also be eased.

• Car Seats

Forty-five years ago in Los Angeles we started to see the dynamic expansion of a modern freeway system, and with it, people sitting in their cars for long stretches going longer distances to get places. With this development I soon began treating people with what I called "commuter back."

When backache continues without addressing the cause of the problem, it can lead to arthritis. I would often recommend that patients roll up a towel and insert it between their lower back and the car seat. If people were in traffic longer than an hour, I would have them get out every hour and stretch. That helps to prevent muscle spasm and tension on the vertebrae.

Today, back-friendly car seats reduce the strain and pain from long sessions at the wheel. Nevertheless, many people spend an hour or more in their cars driving to and from work. If you develop any kind of physical strain on the road, try to change the adjustment of your seat or use the rolled towel.

When driving very long distances at one time, try to make periodic stops. Get out of the car. Stretch. Walk around the vehicle a few times. If you don't mind the stares, do some knee bends alongside the car. If you have chronic back pain, I recommend stopping every half-hour. Otherwise, every hour will do.

Over the years, I have encountered many cases of sciatic pain caused when drivers sit on thick wallets stuffed in their back pockets. I remember one patient in my early days of practice who had bad pain and we couldn't figure what was causing the problem until we realized it was his wallet. Sitting on a thick wallet can create structural stress, chronic pain, and the risk of arthritis. So men, please remove the wallets from your back pockets when you are sitting or driving for long spells.

• **Airline Seats**

Are you a frequent flier? Does your work regularly take you up into the friendly skies in aircraft with notoriously unfriendly seats? Even first class and business seats can be a chronic pain in the neck, back, and butt if you fly often enough.

Contrary to the advertisements, airline seats are possibly the world's worst. I speak from experience: I fly a lot.

I tell my patients who fly to get out of their seats at least once every half-hour and stretch. This can be done standing alongside the seat. If your seat belt must remain fastened for any length of time, do some stretching exercises in your seat.

Here is a simple one that will relieve some of the muscle and ligament strain in the low back area: Bend your head forward and down, between your knees, and hold the position for a few minutes. Then, sit up and raise your knees to your chest, one at a time, holding the position for a few moments.

the bra connection

You would never make the connection, but a pendulous breast can contribute to arthritis in the neck and upper back. I have observed large-breasted patients develop arthritic degeneration and pain of the spine in the lower neck and upper back as a result of inadequate support of the breasts.

Regularly going braless or wearing a flimsy bra can lead to sagging breasts and spinal degeneration in the upper back. This frequently develops into an unsightly curvature known as widow's hump, or kyphosis. Not only does it look unattractive, but it is painful as well. This is more likely to happen to large-breasted women than they might realize.

Pain can start while a woman is in her mid-twenties and peak to an intolerable level by age forty.

Some large-breasted individuals who are sensitive about their breast size tend to pull in their breasts and hunch up. This can result in kyphosis and pain.

You can strengthen the upper back muscles and help prevent the development or progression of this condition by performing a set of "butterflies" with light weights. The weights can be dumbells or anything that fits comfortably in your hands. While standing, hold one weight in each hand against the middle of your chest. Now move each hand forward at the same time and then outward to the sides at shoulder height. Move them from your chest to this extended position with a 1-2 count. Now, bring them back slower to the starting position with a 1-2-3-4 count. Do three sets of ten repetitions daily.

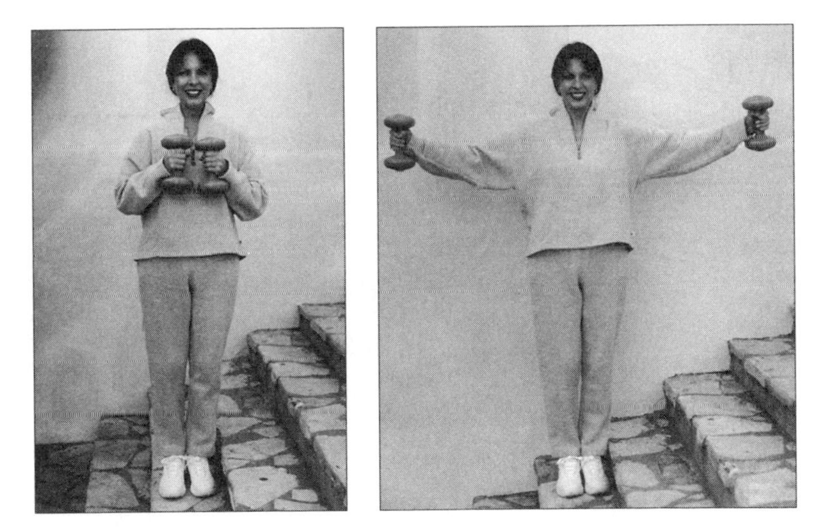

BUTTERFLIES

The breasts should always be supported by a well-built bra with a wide shoulder strap (one inch or more). Save the narrow-strap models for dates or special occasions. Narrow straps can cause chronic pain because they cut into the trapezius muscles, which lie between the shoulder and neck, and irritate the suprascapular nerve, a major nerve in the area. Your daily bra should also have a solid, padded lower band. Large-breasted women in particular should wear a sturdy bra.

If you are an active runner or participate in athletic programs, be sure to use sports bras with solid support, even if you are small- or medium-breasted. This prevents bouncing of the breasts and damage to Cooper's ligament, which connects the breasts and the chest wall. The bouncing action also pulls on muscles, cutting off blood supply and traumatizing adjacent joints. I have treated many women who suffer from pain just because they prefer a natural, braless look when exercising.

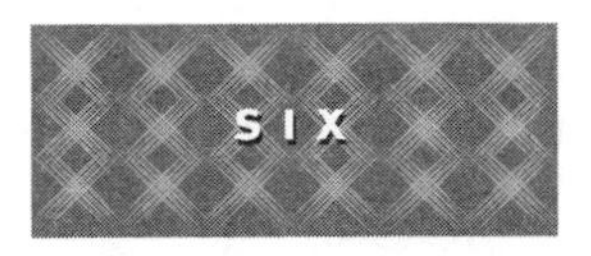

Protect Your Joints after Injury

Experts now believe injuries to joints represent a far more serious risk for osteoarthritis than previously thought, and that injury even in early life often translates to degeneration in later years. Any trauma, they say, that upsets the stability of the joint structure, such as fractures, or tears in the ligaments and soft tissue holding facing bones in place, leads to arthritis in a high percentage of cases.

Obviously, we all attempt to prevent accidents as much as possible in our daily lives, but accidents do happen. However, if you injure a joint you can take concrete steps to prevent, delay, or minimize arthritis.

Trauma to a joint can lead to cartilage breakdown, the fracturing of connective tissue links, the rupture of small capillaries, muscle spasm, and calcium buildup.

Osteoarthritis almost always develops after severe joint injury. But even a minor injury, if ignored, may create conditions for degeneration over the long haul. Enough microtrauma to the knee joint, for instance, can eventually lead to degenerative arthritis.

whiplash

One of the most common injuries in our motorized world is whiplash. Intense forces, generated by rear-end automobile accidents, are transferred to the neck in a rapid acceleration-deceleration action, causing damage to bone and soft tissue. Resultant whiplash disorders run up a huge $29 billion medical bill in the United States alone every year.

No long-term studies have been conducted to determine a connection between whiplash injury and osteoarthritis in the neck. Researchers say it is tricky to do so because osteoarthritis develops anyway with age, and symptoms can be caused by a variety of risk factors. Moreover, some individuals with arthritis in the neck have no symptoms and some with symptoms have no X ray evidence of arthritis.

In my pain practice I have observed countless cases of serious whiplash develop over many years into arthritic and painful degeneration of the vertebral joints in the neck. I have also seen this type of injury lead to disk degeneration and calcium buildup. Often this is due to the rupture of small capillaries in the neck. The tiny amount of blood spilling into adjacent tissues creates a low-grade irritation and a gradual deposit of calcium. Accompanying injury to tendons and ligaments in the neck from a whiplash also contributes to irregular stresses and strains that promote the degenerative process.

After a serious whiplash injury, where symptoms last beyond two or three weeks, I suggest an aggressive healing program to my patients. This includes physical therapy as well as saline solutions into "trigger points" of tenderness in the neck. The injections break up these painful knots, increase blood flow, and reduce inflammation and muscle spasm. The strategy is to deter a chronic problem and the development of calcium deposits.

I also recommend to whiplash patients that they wear the soft cervical collar, open end to the front, whenever they drive or ride in a car. A collar acts as a chin rest, relaxes the neck muscles, and provides good support for a once-injured neck. More important, it reduces the degree of potential damage to the neck in case of a subsequent rear-end accident. I am always concerned about an increased risk of osteoarthritis from a second accident to an already injured neck. Most of my patients won't go to the trouble, but some don't mind doing it.

Some car manufacturers, such as Volvo and SAAB, have recently developed special antiwhiplash car seats with advanced head restraint features. According to Marc White, executive director of the Physical Medicine Research Foundation in Vancouver, experimental data indicates that these added safety systems reduce potential for injury from whiplash. His nonprofit organization, which studies methods to reduce disability and impairment from soft-tissue injuries, is investigating how these seats translate to actual injury reduction on the road.

These types of protective seats are also being installed in some car models by other manufacturers in Europe, Japan, and the United States. The Insurance Corporation of British Columbia is one of the first insurers to recognize the effectiveness of these seats by offering a one-time discount on premiums to motorists who buy cars equipped with them.

sports injuries and arthritis

Bodies are just not made to put up with what we ask them to do.

DICK BUTKUS, FORMER CHICAGO BEAR LINEBACKER

Years ago, I was a consultant to the Denver Broncos and Dallas Cowboys professional football teams. Football, and a number of other sports, are linked to a higher incidence of degenerative arthritis. By watching the action up close and seeing slow motion films it became quite clear to me why this is so. The joints of these athletes repeatedly absorb tremendous blows as well as powerful torsional impact forces. Either through acute trauma or severe wear and tear, the stage is set for arthritis down the line.

Sports injury prevention is an important and doable strategy. Obviously, in whichever sport you participate, there are certain precautions to follow. Be sure to do so, not just for minimizing injury in the present but for protecting yourself against suffering in the future.

Important prevention steps include warm-ups and cool-downs (see next chapter on exercise), strengthening routines, and the use of the right equipment. These measures help you avoid joint injuries and damage to ligaments and other soft tissue, all of which increase the risk of osteoarthritis.

It is also important to treat an injury—whether from sports or any other activity—as quick as possible. Exercising or working through pain may be the macho thing to do, but it is not in your long-term interest. If you have pain or injury, use common sense. If you are an elite athlete, or a professional athlete being paid to play even when injured, you will likely pay a price later on.

Joe Namath, the 1970s Hall of Fame quarterback, is a prime example of the price that pros pay. He ended up with arthritis in multiple joints.

Recently *People* magazine carried an article on Bart Conner, the American gymnast who won two Olympic gold medals in 1984. Today, at forty-two, he suffers from painful osteoarthritis, well before the age most people develop symptoms. He was diagnosed with arthritis when he was in his mid-twenties, even prior to his gold medal performances. Of course, most people don't punish and injure their bodies like gymnasts. Connor has pain now even when doing nothing more strenuous than household chores. "It hurts to bend down and pull weeds in my yard," the former Olympian said.

"Athletes very commonly have osteoarthritis," added John Klippel, M.D., medical director of the Arthritis Foundation. Athletes have increased risk for premature osteoarthritis because of injury as well as repetitive strain. As I discussed in chapter 5, repetitive strain injury in many occupations increases the risk of arthritic degeneration. And athletics, as an occupation, is no exception. Athletes repeatedly twist and strain certain joints, subjecting them to overuse and microtrauma. Sandy Koufax, the great baseball pitcher for the Los Angeles Dodgers in the 1960s, was forced to abbreviate his brilliant career because of an arthritic elbow.

I once had a patient who I treated from the time he was a kid pitcher in Little League up through his playing days in college. As a youngster, the stress on his elbow developed into tendinitis. By his college years, he already had arthritis in the joint.

Baseball pitching is an activity that generates unilateral strain, that is, stressing joints in a particular side of the body. Bowling, golf, and tennis are other popular sports where one side of the body is used much more than the other.

Rotation of an unstable back, as when swinging a golf club, can lead to pain in the low back area. If you stay in good shape by consistent aerobic exercise of some type, the unilateral stress forces will be less apt to create problems.

Arthritis Prevention Starts with Kids

Youngsters in organized kids sports need to receive proper instruction on the biomechanics of their activities and the importance of protective equipment.

Using bats that are too heavy, for instance, can lead to elbow, shoulder, neck, and back problems. You may think this has nothing to do with arthritis. But the potential for arthritis starts when you are born and moving your joints.

If youngsters get into the habit of doing things correctly when they are young, they can help prevent or minimize pain when they are older.

Research says this about athletic activity and arthritis:

- Sports, especially at a high level, raise the arthritis risk considerably, compared to the general population. "Modern elite sport imposes colossal demands upon the performer" and "a heavy price in terms of an early onset of degenerative joint disease," one researcher wrote.
- In particular, sports that generate more acute joint injuries, including damage to the ligaments, joint capsule, menisci, and muscles, increase the risk of degenerative change. Such damage is common

in body contact sports; court sports such as basketball, tennis, and squash; and winter sports such as skiing and skating.

- Competitive sports, as compared to recreational activities, are associated with a higher risk of osteoarthritis. These include football, soccer, rugby, baseball pitching, volleyball, and weightlifting.

- A Swedish study in 1998 found that up to 87 percent of patients with meniscus and cruciate ligament injuries of the knee develop degenerative changes within ten to twenty years. Athletes commonly incur such injuries.

  The two cruciate ligaments form an X behind the kneecap and keep the joint from moving too far forward or backward. Torn ligaments are difficult to repair, leaving the knee less stable and at greater risk for further injury.

  The meniscus is a unique cartilage tissue in the knee that provides an extra layer of protection against the constant forces of jarring pressures and twisting motions. Torn menisci are the cause of many knee surgeries.

- Researchers in Finland analyzed hospital admissions involving former athletes and nonathletes between 1970 and 1990. They looked specifically at osteoarthritis of the hip, knee, and ankle joints. The athlete group comprised 2,049 males who had represented the country in international events from 1920 to 1965.

  Athletes doing endurance, mixed, and power sports* were all found to be at higher risk of requiring hospital care and longer treatment for arthritis of the weight-bearing joints than nonathletes. "Mixed and power sports lead to increased admissions for premature osteoarthritis, but in endurance athletes the admissions are at an

---

* The endurance athletes were long-distance runners and cross-country skiers. Athletes involved in mixed sports played soccer, ice hockey, or basketball, or participated in track-and-field events such as sprinting and middle-distance running, jumping, and hurdling. Power sports included boxing, weightlifting, and throwing (e.g., hammer, javelin, shot put, and discus).

older age," wrote Urho M. Kujala, M.D., of the Helsinki Research Institute for Sports and Exercise Medicine.

arthritis and weight training

The Finnish study tells us that elite weightlifters have a higher risk of developing osteoarthritis at a younger age. To find out more about this I contacted Fred Hatfield, Ph.D., a Connecticut competitor-author and president of the International Sports Sciences Association. Hatfield has set some thirty world power-lifting records and written many books on bodybuilding, sports training, and sports nutrition. At the age of forty-five, he set a world record of 1,014 pounds for the squat.

Today, at fifty-eight, he admits to minor aches but no significant arthritic symptoms. He says X rays show only a slight amount of degeneration in the lower spine.

"Most elite-level weightlifters stay in competition for about ten years and then drop out," says Hatfield. "Afterward, if they continue to lift, they probably follow a recreational routine that is not as intense or damaging to their bodies. It is the individuals who hang in there and lift heavy for thirty or forty years who have an increased risk of osteoarthritis."

Even though, as he admits, "I hung around much longer and lifted heavier than anybody had ever done at my age," Hatfield believes he has protected himself through a careful approach to lifting. "I have always treated this as a science and been very precise in my movements," he says. "I took no unnecessary chances. I developed a solid foundation before I ever lifted heavy weights. So I rarely became injured. Most of the lifters I have known over the years have thrown caution to the wind for the sake of trying to impress or outdo other guys in the gym."

Hatfield believes that two other factors have also helped him.

"First, I may have little genetic predisposition to osteoarthritis, although one can never know that for sure," he says. "Second, I have also followed an extremely careful diet and, for the last fifteen years, have taken a high amount of antioxidant supplements. Even though the research has not definitively proven the connection, I believe there is an involvement of free-radical activity in the degeneration of joints."

Recreational weight training, among both men and women, has become popular in recent years. To what degree does this activity contribute to osteoarthritis? One would think that pumping iron on a regular basis would generate constant microtrauma and irregular forces to the joints and heighten the risk. Unfortunately, there is no research to give us an answer.

"But poor weight-training techniques, practiced over months and years, can exacerbate an arthritic condition," says Hatfield.

In his opinion, the most damaging technique is "attacking a muscle from different angles," a common routine with a combination of several different exercises to develop a particular muscle. In this practice, a joint is forced outside a normal range of motion, traumatizing connective tissue and other soft tissue associated with the joint.

"Irregular pressures and wear on the joints result, which probably accelerates the onset of osteoarthritis," he adds. Shoulders, hips, and knees are likely most affected by this practice.

"On the positive side, weight training makes the bones denser and far less susceptible to injury," says Hatfield. "The skeletal structure adapts to the stress of weight bearing exercise by becoming more dense. This, in turn, will reduce, delay, or even prevent osteoporosis."

Hatfield urges bodybuilders, weightlifters, and power lifters to follow a good diet and use antioxidant supplements to help prevent symptoms of premature aging.

how to speed healing after injury

Whether they were injured by car accidents, occupational mishaps, or sports, I have treated thousands of patients for post-trauma pain and then observed over many years how a once-injured joint frequently becomes prematurely arthritic. For this reason, I generally take an aggressive therapeutic approach to injuries in an attempt to prevent or minimize the development of osteoarthritis.

Obviously, the first thing after injury is to seek appropriate medical attention. If you haven't already done so, be sure to see a physician for any lingering pain following an injury.

My advice to patients includes the following measures to speed up the healing process:

RICE

Usually the standard RICE prescription works well to take care of a minor injury. RICE stands for rest, ice, compression, and elevation. Obviously for major injuries you will be under medical supervision.

Anytime a joint is injured, apply ice during the first twenty-four hours to reduce inflammation. For two weeks or so afterward, or until pain is gone, repeated application of hot moist packs help to bring healing nutrients to the injured area. Don't use dry heat.

Arnica

This, the best known of all homeopathic medicines, is fabulous as a first-aid remedy for major or minor injury, bruising, and inflammation. It produces significant relief of pain and inflammation and also strengthens connective tissue. I have recommended it to many patients. I believe its actions can reduce the potential for a joint injury to lead to arthritis.

You will find arnica in pellet form at the health food store. Buy it at the 30C strength and take it several times a day for a week. For double-barreled relief, purchase arnica gel as well and apply it to the affected joint.

Arnica is so widely accepted today that even plastic surgeons prescribe it before and after operations to reduce inflammation and bleeding.

If you are involved in an activity that you suspect is creating chronic minor trauma to the joints, you can also take arnica periodically for a preventive effect.

Massage and Acupuncture

These methods help break up muscle spasm and increase blood flow to the affected area. See chapter 16 for more details on massage and acupuncture.

Nutrition

As a result of treating thousands of athletes over the years, I developed a high regard for good nutrition as a major contributor to both injury prevention and recovery. If you overlook nutrition, you get hurt more often and just don't heal as fast.

I have treated many athletes, for instance, who ate very poorly and who seemed prone to hamstring and calf pulls, muscle cramps, low back problems, and rotator cuff disorders. They primarily ate fast food with too much salt, sugar, and fat, all of which tend to slow down healing. They didn't ingest enough minerals to prevent pulls and cramps.

For anyone putting a body under the excess stress of training and competition, eating junk food is a sure ticket to malnourishment and injury. If you are an athlete, or a fitness buff, you *must* eat a diet that provides high-quality nutrition. Supplementation is very beneficial but you cannot eat junk food, pop down a handful of vitamins, and still expect to succeed. Eating junk on a regular basis erodes the effort to develop maximum energy, strength, and fitness. It's like building a house on quicksand. Sooner or later it will catch up with you.

I recall the case of a patient who had logged thousands and thousands of miles over decades of daily running. But he couldn't care less about what he ate. By the time he was fifty-five, he was arthritic, losing his teeth, and was overall in bad physical shape.

As far as nonathletes are concerned, younger people can often get away with eating poorly, but as they age the body is less forgiving. I have treated many nonathlete patients who heal very slowly due to poor eating habits.

Most people are inactive while recuperating from injury. That calls for a calorie-restrictive diet and extra care in avoiding unnecessary fat. Some fat is necessary for the healing process, but you will get all you need from a good diet of vegetables, complex carbohydrates, fowl, and fish.

Fast-food restaurants should be off limits to anyone recuperating from injury. A typical fast-food meal is 50 percent fat.

Nutritional Supplements

A supplement regimen can play a major role in both the prevention and the healing of injuries and starts with the use of a quality high-potency multiple vitamin and mineral formula. Among the supplements I consider the most beneficial are the following:

Vitamin C: People recovering from injuries, including the trauma of surgery, use up vast amounts of vitamin C. This is because collagen is the tissue formed from clots created at wound and surgery sites. Vitamin C is absolutely essential in the formation of strong collagen, the fibrous protein that is also a major component of cartilage.

Drs. Emmanuel Cheraskin and W. M. Ringsdorf, Jr., both formerly of the University of Alabama–Birmingham and coauthors of *The Vitamin C Connection* (Bantam, 1984), say there is no doubt that the vitamin speeds healing. Their research shows that from 500 to 3,000 milligrams daily cuts recovery time by as much as 75 percent in many situations.

Preventively, I have found that high doses of vitamin C keep down the incidence of strains, sprains, muscle problems, tendinitis, and other soft-tissue damage among athletes.

Magnesium: This prodigious mineral takes part in some three hundred enzymatic activities in the body, so it's smart never to be deficient. Supplemental magnesium helps prevent chronic muscle cramping (often a sign of magnesium deficiency) and helps heal cartilage injuries.

Supplementation can start with 200 milligrams daily and be increased to 400 milligrams. Take in divided doses with meals.

Magnesium deficiency is widespread. That's because people don't eat enough green, leafy vegetables, a rich source of magnesium. Moreover, processing of grains into refined products (for example, so-called enriched wheat and white rice) severely depletes their magnesium content. Freezing and cooking of vegetables contribute to further losses. The little magnesium most of us have left in the body is burned up through stress.

Zinc: Any event that involves breakdown or rapid turnover of cells—as in injury or surgery—causes the body to excrete up to five times the normal amount of zinc. According to many studies, extra zinc speeds healing. Zinc is rushed to the site of injury to participate directly in the regrowth of damaged tissue. Surgical incisions close up cleaner and faster when zinc is plentiful. The mineral also bolsters the immune system and helps prevent infections.

Zinc deficiency, like magnesium, is commonplace. The use of chemical fertilizers has rendered agricultural soil zinc deficient in many states. Zinc is also lost during food processing.

Take 50 to 150 milligrams of zinc daily in divided doses during the healing period.

B complex: Two members of the B complex family of vitamins are particularly important healers. Vitamin B6 is one. It cuts down the edema of an injury and helps transport damaged tissue out of the system. It is also a strategic factor in protein metabolism, ensuring that more protein becomes available for tissue repair and growth.

Niacin (vitamin B3) is a vasodilator, that is, it opens the blood vessels for a strong flow of circulation—important for tissue repair. You probably will get enough of these two important B factors in a high-potency multivitamin.

Amino acids: A multiple amino-acid formula ensures an adequate supply of optimally assimilable protein. Amino acids are the components of protein. A supplement can be particularly helpful when caloric intake is restricted during any period of injury recovery. L-ornithine and L-arginine, two amino acids that stimulate growth-hormone release, play important roles in the wound-healing process. L-arginine, in particular, assists in collagen formation.

Glucosamine: This now famous joint supplement, known for its ability to reduce the pain of arthritis, may also have particular benefit for joint injuries. Glucosamine is a naturally occurring ingredient that contributes to key proteins that bind water in cartilage tissue.

In one European study, sixty-eight athletes with knee-cartilage damage were given 1,500 milligrams of glucosamine daily for forty days, and then 750 milligrams for ninety to one hundred days. Fifty-two had complete resolution of symptoms and resumed full athletic training. After four to five months, athletes were able to train at pre-injury rates. Follow-up examinations twelve months later showed no signs of cartilage damage in any of the athletes.

MSM: This popular natural pain reliever, a source of biologically active sulfur, appears also to speed recovery from injury. In 1999, I collaborated with two Los Angeles–area chiropractors to test its healing effect on acute strain and sprain injuries sustained during athletic activities. The subjects for the experiment were twenty-four individuals who had been injured within thirty days and were receiving similar therapy—routine manipulation, ultrasound, and muscle stimulation.

The patients were randomly divided. Half were given inert placebo pills to take on a daily basis, while the other half were given Lignisul

MSM, a high-quality MSM supplement. The study was done in a "double-blind" fashion, meaning that neither patients nor doctors knew if the pills were placebo or MSM. Only an independent evaluator knew who was getting what. When we "broke the code," the results showed an impressive healing acceleration among the MSM users, as reported both by patients and physicians. The patients on MSM required 40 percent fewer office visits, representing a sizable economic bonus.

MSM is known for anti-inflammatory properties, reduction of pain and muscle spasm, and blood-flow increase. The amount of MSM used in the study was 1,000 milligrams three times daily.

The Pineapple Rx

Put the common pineapple atop your list of healing foods.

Pineapple contains an enzyme called bromelain that contributes to the healing process by breaking down injured tissue.

Best eat the pineapple fresh—within an hour of taking off the husk. If not, the bromelain is prone to oxidize and quickly lose its therapeutic effect.

Eat as much as you can every other day. You'll be surprised at how it speeds recovery.

If you aren't into pineapple, you may want to try bromelain or papain enzyme supplements. Papain is extracted from papayas.

The super healing properties of enzyme supplements have been documented in many studies, which show they cut short hospital stays after surgery and reduce pain and inflammation in a wide variety of injuries.

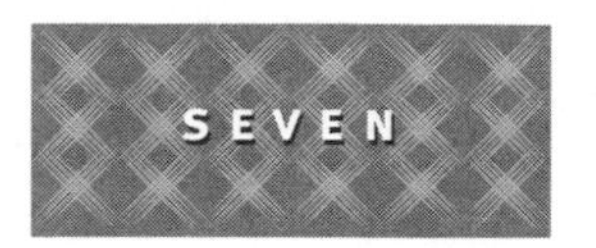

Exercise (but Don't Abuse) Your Joints

Movement is life.

—ARISTOTLE

Of all the causes which conspire to render the life of man short and miserable, none have greater influence than the want of proper exercise.

—WILLIAM BUCHAN, NINETEENTH-CENTURY SCOTTISH PHYSICIAN

I am seventy-five years old. I have no arthritic pain and I move well, yet X rays indicate there is degenerative disk disease in my spine.

I have been exercising routinely since the age of forty-one, when I began running. Before that, I didn't follow any regular exercise routine. I was shocked into exercise by the sudden death of my forty-year-old medical partner from a heart attack. I had no intention of letting that happen to me, so I undertook a vigorous exercise program for my cardiovascular health. With time, I became more aware of the benefits of exercise for the rest of the body, including the joints.

I have since run in two hundred marathons and once even did a hundred-mile run. I have logged a lot of miles. All this exercise, I strongly believe, has helped keep me free of arthritic pain.

I vigorously preach exercise to my patients. If they don't exercise, they usually hear from me. Over the years I developed a reputation for being the exercise doctor. Many patients gravitated to me for an exercise therapy program for their pain conditions or as part of an overall health and prevention approach.

From observing many thousands of patients, it became quite clear that those who exercised not only lived longer lives on average, but looked and felt remarkably better. If these individuals developed arthritis, I observed that they normally had fewer complaints and less pain.

Doing nothing, that is, leading a very sedentary life, appears to contribute to osteoarthritis. This is a very strange concept for a lot of people. If repetitive motion over time wears down the cartilage, as we have seen, how can the opposite, such as sitting at a desk all day and then going home to watch TV for several hours, also lead to osteoarthritis?

We all know that exercise helps the heart, lungs, and blood vessels. Similarly, all my clinical experience and interpretation of the research indicate it helps the joints as well. The key to good prevention appears to be reasonable recreational exercise performed regularly within a comfort zone that puts joints through normal motions, and without the existence of an underlying joint abnormality. Regular exercise outside the comfort zone, and in the presence of joint abnormalities, may contribute to arthritis (see excess exercise later in this chapter).

The saying, use it or lose it, applies to arthritis. That's why exercise is so important. Here's what it does:

- Makes bones stronger by drawing calcium into the bone cells.
- Strengthens muscles, tendons, and ligaments, all of which support, stabilize, and move the joints.
- Lubricates the joints and keeps them pliable. The same lubricating effect prevents pain and flare-ups for those who already have arthritis. Cartilage tissue has no blood supply per se, so the joint capsule and cartilage tissue rely on movement to receive essential nutrients and oxygen and be cleansed. Movement thus works like a pump—bringing in needed supplies and flushing out wastes. At the Univer-

sity of Heidelberg, in Germany, researchers recently developed sophisticated microcatheters that permitted, for the first time, measurement of the amount of increased oxygen supplied to knee-joint tissue by exercise. They found that exercise raises the oxygen pressure to a much greater degree among nonarthritics than among arthritic patients. An arthritic knee, they point out, contains "disturbance factors" that interfere with cartilage nutrition. This scientific work provides strong direct evidence for the value of exercise in ensuring maximum delivery of vital substances to the joint.

exercise and osteoarthritis—a researcher's perspective

Steve Blair, P.E.D., director of research at the internationally famous Cooper Institute in Dallas, is one of the world's leading experts on the relationship of exercise to health. He has followed the lifestyle and health status of thousands of patients who have visited the clinic, founded by Kenneth Cooper, M.D., the "father of aerobic exercise."

Q: *Can exercise promote osteoarthritis, and if so, which exercises?*

A: *It is pretty clear from occupational studies that you can cause arthritic changes in a joint by repetitive, strenuous motions that create repetitive strain injuries. Jackhammer operators, for instance, develop osteoarthritis in the wrists and shoulders. Clearly, you can do too much.*

Years ago I attended a medical meeting on injuries involving military personnel around the world. I recall two reports on Israeli commandos and U.S. Army rangers who developed arthritis as a result of their extreme training activities. These are supremely fit young men, who may run ten miles before breakfast, then swim, do calisthenics, and later in the day hike for thirty miles carrying a fifty-pound backpack.

While there is considerable osteoarthritis in the U.S. population, I don't think we can attribute much of that to physical activity. When you look at any population overall, a level of activity equivalent to that of military elite troops is virtually nonexistent. In my opinion, the high prevalence of osteoarthritis in the middle-aged and older population cannot really be charged to physical activity.

If you look at athletes who develop arthritis later on, that's another story. You can attribute their joint problems to trauma. Football yields striking examples of traumatized joints.

For osteoarthritis of the hips and knees, researchers have a fairly clear picture that the important risk factors are obesity, gender (women are at greater risk), age, and prior traumatic injury. Injuries incurred from football or other sports will show up as arthritic changes years later. Physical activity per se is not included in this list simply because we don't have any incriminating data.

Q: *Does research show that physical activity really helps prevent osteoarthritis?*

A: *We haven't done the real good epidemiological studies on humans to definitively say yes. I have been asked this question by arthritis experts, and the answer is that we just don't really know how physical activity might be protective. It might be that it is protective, in different amounts and in different people, but as we have just seen, it certainly can be harmful if we are talking about activities that cause strenuous repetitive motion and traumatic injury.*

There is, however, some indirect evidence that it may be protective. There are animal studies showing that exercise generates thicker cartilage, more lubricating fluids, and stronger joints. Surprisingly, we don't have such data on humans. The studies haven't been done. However, this is a direction of research that I will be intensely pursuing in the next few years.

If we are going to recommend physical activity as good health behavior, and we already have national recommendations, we ought to know what the potential risk is for osteoarthritis. I have tried to pin down some of the leading arthritis experts. I have said to them that surely the consensus public-health recommendation for thirty minutes of moderately intense activity a day cannot be harmful. They told me that this is probably so, but even they don't really have the research to back it up.

I personally believe that the regular amount of nontraumatic exercise being widely recommended is very likely to be protective. I base that on logic. Human beings were designed to be endurance animals. It seems unlikely to me that we can wear out our knees and hip joints with thirty minutes of walking. I believe that ultimately the research will prove this to be the case.

Q: *Does physical activity help in the treatment of osteoarthritis?*

A: *There are data on physical activity for people with osteoarthritis, and particularly of the knee. I wish we had larger numbers and more joints covered in these studies.*

In one recent study, researchers at Wake Forest University took about three hundred elderly people with osteoarthritis of the knee and randomly divided them into three different programs: health education, aerobic walking, or strength training. The participants were followed for eighteen months. Both exercise activities were found to be beneficial. Neither program affected the status of the disease, that is, there was no cure or regression, but the people reported less pain, better mobility and quality of life, and greater function in general. The study was impressive in showing the amount of benefit in this group of people.

The general view in the medical community and among the public is that walking is helpful. People will say that they can't walk because they have arthritis in the knee. The fact is they will feel better. It won't cure the arthritis but they will be better off.

I am convinced that exercise of the proper type and amount, and under some medical guidance at the beginning, is clearly beneficial for people with arthritis.

exercise doesn't have to be strenuous

"No pain, no gain" is a popular saying among the ultrafitness and bodybuilding crowd. For our purposes, pain is definitely not on the agenda. We are, after all, trying to prevent pain.

An effective exercise program need not be strenuous. Too rigorous a program often scares people away from doing any type of leisure physical activity. What's needed is a regular and moderate program that's good for the heart and at the same time good for the joints.

In general, the best exercise (and the most inexpensive) for arthritis prevention is walking. You want an activity in which the feet strike the ground, creating a natural impact effect that is transferred to the joints. Although I have been an avid runner for years, running is not necessary for fitness and arthritis prevention. Walking is enough. It's ideal for the anatomy. We evolved on this type of locomotion.

I have had one patient for fifty years who is my age and walks every day. He is not an enthusiastic walker, but he does it without fail. He has had a number of health problems over the years, but I am convinced that walking has kept them to a minimum.

I have recommended walking to thousands of patients and I feel hugely successful when I convince them to walk briskly for a half-hour or more a day. Actually, I prefer an hour.

But maybe walking doesn't appeal to you. No problem. Today, there are so many different exercise opportunities. The important thing is to find something that inspires you, ideally, an activity that you can incorporate into your lifestyle. Join an exercise group for the additional social contact, pursue a fitness program at a gym, or do it yourself. Just do something.

Swimming, cycling, and cross-country skiing are also excellent conditioners. When the season or weather doesn't allow a particular outdoor activity, go inside to utilize a treadmill, stationary bike, or NordicTrack machine.

In the early days of my career, physicians who recommended exercise to patients simply picked one activity or another. One activity would favor certain joints and muscles; a different activity would favor others. As I later learned, an even better and safer overall approach is cross-training. I subsequently began recommending to patients that they alternate their activities. By this I mean a personally appealing blend of walking, cross-country skiing, bicycling, and swimming. One activity on one day, a different one the next, or several different exercises in one day. Whatever formula works best, try to include some walking or cross-country skiing. I do believe that our bodies benefit from the natural impact these activities generate.

People like variety. Patients tell me it keeps them from becoming bored. My experience suggests that those who cross-train may have a much lower risk of developing arthritis than those who focus on one activity. Different groups of muscles are being utilized and strengthened, instead of all the strain and demand being exerted continually on one set of muscles.

And take some time to work in a light weight-training routine as part of your exercise plan.

Fitness expert Bob Delmonteque, N.D., makes the point that a simple, regular, light weight-resistant program makes a great contribution to overall fitness as well as joint health.

"Just a few minutes with light weights can tone and strengthen the muscles, ligaments, and tendons that support the joints," says Delmonteque, who has coached the likes of Marilyn Monroe, Gloria Swanson, Eric Braedon, Paul Newman, Matt Dillon, Clark Gable, John Wayne, and astronaut John Glenn. "Done regularly, light weights will boost flexibility, lubricate the joints, and prevent muscle and other soft tissue weakness that could increase your risk of arthritis."

At age eighty-one, Delmonteque is widely regarded as the most physically fit individual for his age. He follows a rigorous cross-training program and still lifts heavy weights.

"My program is too hard for most people sixty years younger than me," he says. "But you don't need to go to my level. Just find a program you enjoy doing for the long haul because it is going to help your joints, heart, emotions, and each and every part of you. And I believe contribute to your longevity as well."

THE ARTHRITIS PREVENTION EXERCISE PROGRAM

Before embarking on this or any exercise program, consult with your physician. It is prudent to undergo a thorough checkup if you haven't exercised for a long period of time, are over age thirty-five, or have a health problem.

Always begin modestly, without straining yourself. Work yourself up to a level where you are slightly sweating and puffing.

Check your pulse—a measure of your heart rate—as a guide. In the early 1970s, I participated in the development of the target heart-rate formula that has since become a widely used standard for obtaining maximum aerobic benefits from exercise.

The simple formula is this:

1. Subtract your age from 220.
2. Take 60 to 80 percent of the remainder. That number is your goal—your heart-beat target zone. If you are a beginner at exercise, take 60 percent, or even 50 percent if you are in poor physical shape. If you are a regular exerciser, take 70 percent. If you are highly trained and fit, take 80 percent or more. Let's say you are fifty years old and exercise fairly regularly. You would apply the formula like this: 220 minus 50 = 170 × 70 percent = 119 heart beats per minute.
3. Try to reach your target and stay in the zone for a good portion of your exercise session. If you exercise for twenty minutes, aim for about ten minutes in the zone. If you exercise for a half-hour, try for about fifteen minutes in the zone. For a forty-five-minute workout, stay in the zone for about a half-hour.

Be flexible. Don't allow yourself to feel challenged, breathless, or stressed. After exercise, check your pulse again. In the beginning, your return to a "baseline" (pre-exercise) heart rate should not take more than ten minutes. As you develop cardiovascular fitness, the recovery time will be much faster, even within two or three minutes.

Always limber up for about two minutes before you exercise. You want to raise the temperature in your muscles and tendons, and loosen them up, lubricate your joints, and gradually put your heart into a higher gear. If you go out fast all at once, you load up your muscles with lactic acid, a waste product that can cause cramping and aching.

If your exercise is walking, warm up with some slow, gentle strolling. If you are swimming, take a couple of minutes of slow, gentle stroking.

For most people, stretching is unnecessary before exercise. If, however, you are going all out and extending yourself beyond a usual range of motion, lengthening and loosening the muscles beforehand is advisable.

In general, stretching is most important afterward as a cool-down practice to relax the particular muscles that have been used the most during exercise. Take more time to do this—six to eight minutes, if possible. Contracted muscles lead to diminished blood flow to the joints. If you swim laps, gear down with a few easy laps. By not stretching after exercise (vigorous or otherwise), muscles can go into what we call rebound spasm.

How Much Should You Exercise?

Exercise at least every other day and, if possible, every day.

walking

- Start with twenty minutes.
- Increase to a half-hour each session for another week or so.
- If you are comfortable and have the time, move up to forty-five minutes or an hour.

- Increase your speed gradually. The average person can walk about a mile in a half-hour at the start. With the conditioning gained within a few weeks, you should be able to cover the same distance in twenty minutes. If you really step up your speed and push, you can do the mile in fifteen minutes. A ten-minute mile walk is very vigorous.

Resources

Sherry Brourman's excellent book *Walk Yourself Well* (Hyperion, 1998) is a great one-stop reference for learning to walk correctly, preventively, and for the elimination of back, neck, shoulder, knee, hip, and other structural pain.

Magazines such as *Walking* (*www.walkingmag.com;* phone: 800-829-5585) and *Walking Connection* (*www.walkingconnection.com;* phone: 800-295-WALK) are fine periodicals dedicated to promoting the art and enjoyment of walking.

cycling

- You have a variety of options: outdoors on a bicycle and indoors on a stationary bike. For individuals with impaired balance, adult tricycles are available.

- Outdoors, ride on a flat surface in the beginning. Indoors, adjust the controls for a flat ride. Save the hills and more strenuous cycling for when you are more conditioned.

- When you start, monitor the state of your legs. You will feel the stress most in the thighs. As soon as the thighs begin feeling fatigued, head for home. If you are on a stationary bike, that's a sign to start slowing down.

- Your initial goal is to ride at a moderate pace (you're huffing a bit) for a half-hour.

- Gradually increase your distance and speed, and if you want the added workout, head for the hills.

- If you have any type of chronic back pain, whether from a disk problem or arthritis, you may want to consider a recumbent bicycle. These bikes look like "lawn chairs on wheels." Your body is supported by a full seat and back rest, as compared to the standard bike, which offers no such support. Your legs are straight forward, pumping the pedals located toward the front end of the bike. Recumbents start in price at around $350. They tend to be more expensive than mass-produced upright bikes because fewer of them are manufactured.

- Just in case you want to know what it takes to be a super cyclist, you are considered a master once you can handle a two-hour ride several times a week at just below a twenty-mile-an-hour pace.

- If you ride outdoors, take all safety precautions—helmets, mirrors, and so forth—to protect your joints, and the rest of you, from mishaps. Consult with a cycling shop.

Resources

Bicycling magazine (*www.bicycling.com;* phone: 800-666-2806) is a popular monthly publication that covers all you need to know about cycling practicalities, equipment, safety, and tours.

swimming

- If you don't know how to swim, or aren't sure about your technique, take some lessons.

- Unless you are a skilled swimmer and can handle the ocean waves, your best bet is to stay in a heated pool. You can pace yourself and set distance goals according to the number of laps you swim.

- Swimming puts less demand on the circulatory system than "land-based" exercise. Unlike in upright exertion, you swim on your back or stomach. Your heart has up to 20 percent more blood in this position, and with less effort it pumps out more blood with each contraction. Thus, in order to get the same aerobic benefit as say rapid walking or cycling, you will have to exercise twice as long in the water as out of it. And you'll have to make it an effort, not just piddling along at a turtle pace.

- In the beginning, swim as far as you can until you feel tired. The distance may be less than one lap of the pool. But no matter. Stop and rest as often as you need. Each time you will be able to go farther.

- Build up over a period of weeks, or even months, to where you can swim for about an hour without stopping. Maintain a pace whereby you are slightly huffing. If you stick to it, you should be able to cover eight hundred or a thousand yards in that time, or up to forty lengths in a twenty-five-yard pool.

- For inexperienced swimmers, I recommend that a "float belt" be worn around the abdomen. The reason for this is to avoid stressing the low back. Beginners typically arch their backs to keep their heads out of the water. This makes breathing easier, but it also puts a strain on the muscles in the low back. Float belts are filled with air. They support your midsection and enable you to swim without arching the back. These devices are available at sporting goods stores.

- You can consider yourself an intermediate swimmer if you can do a thousand yards in less than twenty-five minutes and you are forty to sixty years old. Over sixty, you will probably lose about 1 percent of your speed each year.

Resources

Sports Publications (*www.swiminfo.com;* phone: 800-352-7946) offers books, videos, and magazines on swimming techniques, workouts, and equipment.

cross-training

- Perform different exercises—such as walking, cross-country skiing, swimming, cycling, and weight training—on alternate days, or split your daily workout between two or more activities.
- Indoor exercisers, such as NordicTrack or stationary bicycles, can be used when the weather doesn't permit a particular activity. Health clubs, with their wide variety of exercise machines, are excellent facilities for pursuing a cross-training program.
- Exercise twenty to thirty minutes daily or every other day, and try to build up to an hour.

Resources

Cross-Training for Dummies by Tony Ryan and Martica Heaner (Foster City, CA: IDG Books, 2000).

weight training

- A simple, light weight program to tone up the five major muscle groups in your arms, legs, and upper back is a good starting point.
- If you have no experience with weights, consult with your physician for the name of a sports medicine specialist or physical therapist who can advise you on proper lifting techniques.

Whatever you do, be sure to follow the old saying "Fools rush in where wise men fear to tread." Take it easy with weights. Always start light and just do a few repetitions so as not to develop sore or injured muscles and joints. Don't be in a hurry. Just go slowly, safely, and steadily. Start at a very low and comfortable level of weight and increase your repetitions and weight gradually as you desire.

"Just baby yourself," says Delmonteque. "You're not racing anybody."

- If you belong to a health spa, you have a considerable amount of "iron" and weight-resistant machines at your disposal. You can do the exercises described here with free weights or on the machines. Do whatever is most comfortable for you.

- If you are not a spa member, and want to exercise on your own, purchase a pair of light dumbbells and adjustable ankle weights (two of each) in a sporting goods store. "Depending on your condition and strength, anywhere from two to twenty pounds is a good starting point," advises Delmonteque. "Try the weights in the store to see what you are comfortable with."

- Perform the contraction segment of each repetition to a 1-2 count. Take longer to do the relaxation segment. Use a 1-2-3-4 count for that. "The rhythm and the counting are important," says Delmonteque. "It helps you concentrate on what you are doing and sends messages to the muscles you are working."

- Start with five repetitions of each exercise and very slowly work your way up to twenty or thirty repetitions. It could take several months to build up to that level. Add weight, if you wish, as is comfortable for you.

- ***Curls—Exercise 1.*** Do a set of curls with each arm to tone up the biceps, the muscle at the front of the upper arm. Stand, holding a dumbbell in each hand, with your hands hanging at your sides. With one hand, bring the weight up toward your shoulder. Keep your wrist straight. Then lower the weight. Repeat with the other hand.

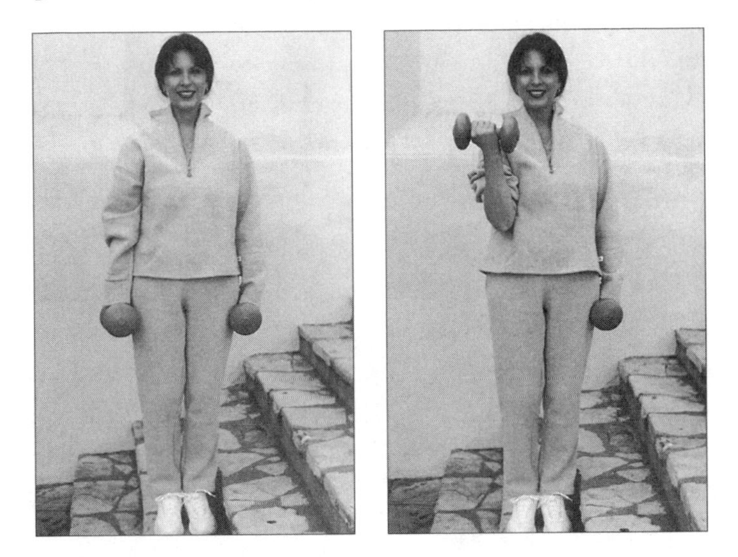

- ***French presses—Exercise 2***. Do a set of French presses with each arm to tone the triceps, located at the back of the upper arm. Start with the elbow fully bent and pointed upward and as close to your head as is comfortable. Raise the weight up in one hand toward the ceiling by unbending your elbow. Then lower it. Repeat with the other hand.

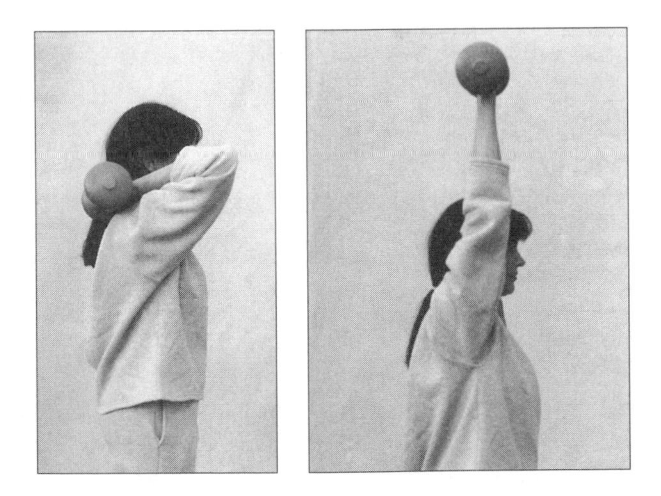

- ***Presses—Exercise* 3.** Do a set of presses with dumbbells to strengthen your shoulders and trapezius, the big muscle in your upper back and neck. Perform the exercise either standing or sitting. Hold the weights in front of you, palms facing forward, at shoulder level. Press both weights simultaneously upward and overhead, fully extending your arms. Then lower them to the start position.

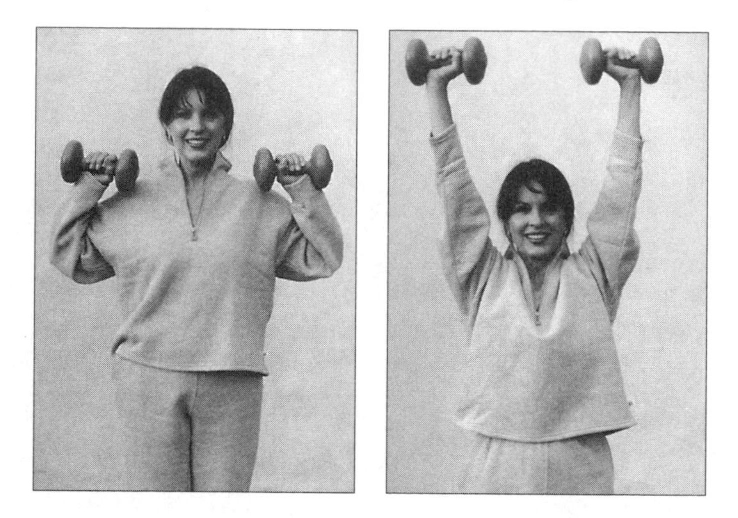

- ***Leg curls—Exercise* 4.** Do a set of leg curls to tone up the hamstrings, the big muscle at the back of the thigh. Attach the ankle weights. Lie, stomach down, on a bench or the floor, with your legs extended so that you are in a straight line from head to toe. Bend your knee, raise one foot, and bring it up and forward toward your butt. Return it to the starting position. Do this maneuver one leg at a time.

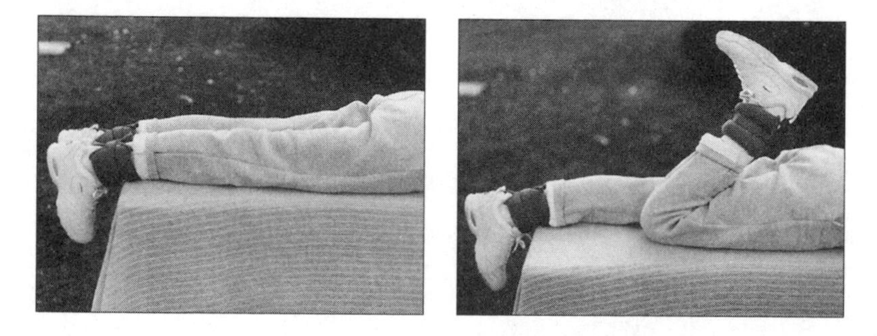

- ***Leg extensions—Exercise 5.*** Do a set of leg extensions with each leg to tone the quadriceps, the big muscle in the front of the thigh. Weak quads can lead to arthritis in the knee, particularly among women. Studies have shown that among aging women, weakness of the quadriceps often precedes the development of osteoarthritis of the knee. The muscle helps hold the patella—the kneecap—in position. When the muscle atrophies, the kneecap tends to "float" out of position and lose stability. This subjects the knee to constant low-grade trauma, the result of irregular forces exerted by other bones, muscles, and tendons involved with the knee.

  Keeping the quadriceps strong helps prevent arthritis of the knee. A simple exercise called the leg extension can accomplish this very easily.

  For this simple exercise, you will need light ankle weights if you don't do it on a machine in the gym. As a substitute to ankle weights, you can use an old purse filled with rocks or cans of food. Men will probably want to use a heavier ankle weight than women.

  Sit on the edge of a table, bar stool, or bench. Strap the weights around your ankles. If you are using a purse, you can hang it from your pointed toe.

  Start with your knees bent at a 90-degree angle and your feet dangling down. Refer to the photograph. Exercise one leg at a time.

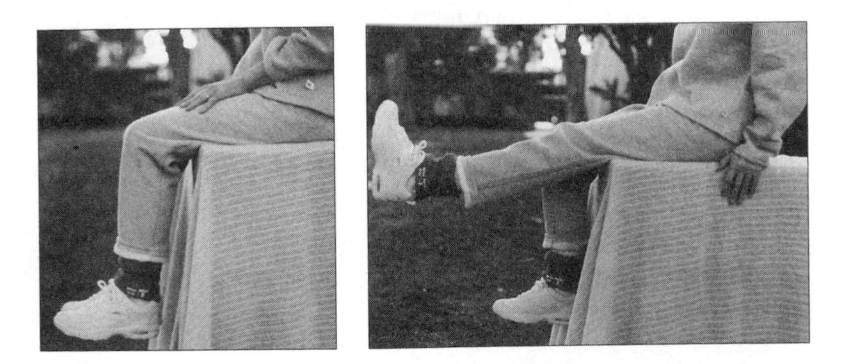

To a count of 1-2, straighten the weighted foot upward and outward so that the knee is locked. The leg is now fully extended and parallel to the floor. Hold it there for a second or two.

Release and bend the knee, and slowly allow the lower leg to return to the starting position. The return movement should be done to a 1-2-3-4 count. The major strengthening effect occurs when you do the return movement slowly, not, as most people might think, when you lift the leg with the weight.

Start with two pounds, or whatever weight is comfortable for you, and gradually increase it if you would like to develop your quadriceps even more. If it is comfortable, increase to ten pounds. For each leg, perform three sets of ten repetitions daily or every other day. Take a moment to rest, if needed, between each set.

For women, one of the "side benefits" of this strengthening exercise is an attractive firming up of the thigh muscle.

about running and arthritis

For many years, physicians involved in sports medicine, and particularly those like myself taking part in the medical support of marathon races, questioned whether long-distance running and training increase the risk of osteoarthritis in the weight-bearing joints. The question was studied comprehensively by Peter Jokl, M.D., director of the Yale Sports Medicine Center, who found that running per se will not cause arthritis. However, if a person already has arthritis, running can make it worse. Or, if structural abnormalities are present in the lower extremities, there is potential for joint damage.

I love running. I have been doing it for thirty years, and have served as president of the American Running Association. Nevertheless, I don't recommend running to my patients.

Here is why: Running causes about half the injuries treated by sports-medicine specialists. The injuries include stress fractures of the feet and lower legs, ankle sprains, heel spurs and inflamed Achilles tendons, shinsplints, knee problems, and damage to the disks in the lower back. Some of these injuries have the potential to increase the risk of arthritis. It is not the running itself that contributes to arthritis, but the injuries. So why look for trouble, when walking is much less demanding and traumatic.

For women, there is another consideration here. The female pelvic alignment may not always support risk-free running activity. Compared to men, a woman's shape is frequently associated with an angulation of the femur (thigh) bones that can create extra stress on the hips and knees during running. This extra stress, in turn, might increase the risk of developing osteoarthritis in these joints, particularly the knees. Women have different degrees of femur angulation, making some individuals more vulnerable than others. If you are a woman who likes to run, I recommend consulting with a sports-medicine specialist to determine if your skeletal structure is "runner friendly."

In addition to the injury issue, research shows that 90 percent of people who start running for exercise give it up within six months. In a year's time, less than 5 percent are still running. They find that they develop back or knee problems (women more than men). Or soon they realize that running is a lot of work and getting psyched up for the morning run becomes harder and harder.

Over the years I found that people who started running often traded in their running shoes for walking shoes. Unless you really love running, like I do, there is no sense in doing it.

If you do run for exercise, you must do it properly and avoid common pitfalls that can lead to trouble. I recommend the following:

• Watch Your Step

The patient came into my office limping noticeably. He was a sixty-year-old business executive who had been running regularly for more than a dozen years. His choice of a running route, while interesting from a sightseeing standpoint, was a disaster for his knees. He loved to run on the concrete pathway that zigzags for miles along the Santa

Monica Bay beachfront, winding through beaches filled with bikini-clad beauties, the circus atmosphere of Venice, and the hard bodies of Muscle Beach. It's a scene that draws a heavy traffic of in-line skaters, cyclists, runners, and tourists.

X rays showed extensive osteoarthritis in the knee joints.

About five years before I had first seen him for knee pain. I advised him at the time to buy the best running shoes, with special supports, and to stop running on concrete.

He bought the good shoes but continued to run on the concrete. For him, and the knees of hundreds of other running enthusiasts I have treated, concrete proved disastrous. We live in an expanding concrete universe but didn't evolve in one. It's a surface not particularly friendly to the human body. Regular running, and even walking, on hard surfaces is an invitation to degenerative arthritis.

Each time you plant your foot on such a surface, you deliver a force throughout your body equal to two and one half times your weight. The spinal column absorbs much of this jolt, and eventually a painful osteoarthritis condition may develop along the spine, or in the knees.

I tell patients better not run at all if you have to run on concrete. You need to find a surface that is more giving . . . and forgiving. Asphalt is much better. It gives. Better yet is a dirt running track at a high school. If it's winter and wet, then run on a treadmill.

In the early days of my running "career," I was unaware of the problem with concrete. Luckily, as I delved deeper into the science of running, I learned the facts and avoided concrete. Given the many miles I have logged, I am convinced that I spared myself a good deal of pain and grief.

If you run on an asphalt surface, such as a street, try to run in the middle, if that is possible. Running on the side of the street is not a good idea, because streets have a curved surface to facilitate water runoff toward the curbs. Running on such an uneven surface can cause irregular wear on the knees.

A flat grassy surface is ideal. However, grassy surfaces tend to be uneven with hidden small holes here and there. That can be hard on the knees and back.

- **Use proper footware**

Running with inadequate shoes can lead to arthritis in the hips, knees, or lower back. The best bet is to go to a store specializing in running equipment and be fitted for shoes.

- **Leg length differences**

Consult with a chiropractor or knowledgeable physician to check out your leg length. Differences between the length of the right and left leg are common. A pronounced difference can cause irregular wear on joints.

- **See a podiatrist**

Have your feet evaluated. Running on fallen arches, pronated or deformed toes, can contribute to arthritis in the feet, knees, hips, and back. A podiatrist can advise you as to how to compensate for these conditions by using special shoe inserts called orthotics (see page 252).

excess exercise and arthritis

All things in excess bring trouble to men.

—PLAUTUS, ROMAN WRITER

Men have traditionally fallen into the excess trap: If a little exercise is good, more is better. But now, increasingly, women may be overdoing it as well. Man or woman, this increases the potential for arthritis.

Muscles and ligaments become tense. The joints are strained, creating microtrauma. The metabolism of the cartilage is negatively affected.

Moreover, the excess can cause small capillaries to become ruptured, particularly in the area where ligaments attach to the joints. This doesn't produce significant discomfort unless many capillaries are involved. Often the body clears up the damage overnight. But if the tissue is subjected to routine punishment, scar tissue will develop. Scar tissue leads to calcium formation, and this can pave the way for degenerative changes and arthritis.

How do you know if you are exercising too much? I've been asked that question many times.

Your body will tell you. One way it tells you is through persistent discomfort after exercise, anything lasting more than a minute or two. Another indicator is how you feel the next morning. If you wake up with aches and pains in the muscles and joints you exercised the hardest, that means you overdid it. DOMS, or delayed-onset muscle soreness, is an indicator that you are overworking.

If these signs develop, cut back a bit next time. If you want to increase your intensity, do it slowly to a level that doesn't cause the soreness afterward.

It's a different story if you are a professional athlete, weightlifter, or fitness buff seeking to develop muscle. In those cases you are likely looking for the so-called burn, the searing feeling that comes with the intensity needed for muscle hypertrophy (enlargement). However, if the burn lasts for more than a minute or two, or if you have soreness and stiffness the next day, you are really doing too much. You can prevent this by reducing the time involved in the particular exercise.

Over the years I have seen more male patients with joint problems related to excess exercise. But in the last decade I have treated increasing numbers of women involved in intense fitness and bodybuilding programs. Excess use of stair-stepping machines at fitness centers causes numerous knee and lower-back problems. More recently, I have seen quite a few women who practice Tae Bo, a hybrid workout that involves punching and kicking routines. The sudden thrusts of arms and legs can produce capillary rupture and microtrauma to the joints.

Pain specialists routinely see patients with self-inflicted conditions brought about by fitness excesses. These are people who try to get too fit, too firm, or too muscular too soon, or who just do more than their bodies can handle.

As I see it, the problem is dose related. Exercise done at a nonexhausting level enhances the immune system. But if you do too much, you deplete the system. Medication works the same way. A little bit may be beneficial. Too much can make you sick or even kill you.

An experiment conducted with laboratory animals some years ago demonstrated this point. In the study, one group of rodents was run to exhaustion and a second group put through a lesser ordeal. Afterward, all animals were exposed to a virus. The results: rampant infections among the first group, increased resistance among the second.

I have seen many people get quite sick with anything from hepatitis to the common cold after exhaustive training or marathon races. After runners complete marathons, their immune systems may be shot for weeks.

Moreover, exhaustive physical exercise leads to an excess burden of muscle-fiber destruction that the body cannot repair. The continual stress that intense and repetitive physical activity places on the joints can also cause microtrauma and probably damage to the cartilage.

Here is what the research says about excess exercise and arthritis:

- There is increasing concern that too much physical activity may lead to osteoarthritis.

- Heavy physical activity can be a significant risk factor for knee osteoarthritis in the elderly, particularly among obese individuals. Light and moderate activities do not appear to increase the risk.

- Individuals of all ages can tolerate moderate amounts of exercise without adverse consequences or accelerated development of osteoarthritis.

- The onset of osteoarthritis appears to depend on a variety of factors such as the frequency, intensity, and duration of physical activity; the presence of abnormal joint anatomy or alignment, joint instability, underlying muscle weakness or imbalance; and body weight.

do's and don'ts

The advice on fitness and muscle building is simple. Just go slow. Build up slowly over weeks and months, not days. If you feel any discomfort, stop what you are doing. Be sure that you warm up properly.

Don't be a mindless zealot. I have treated many fitness enthusiasts who rush into a hundred fast push-ups instead of starting low and increasing slowly. They set themselves up for trauma to the elbows and shoulders.

Make sure you follow proper biomechanics for the exercise you are pursuing, and using equipment that fits you. Specialty stores and professional instructors are your best bet for avoiding problems later on. You may be setting yourself up for problems down the line if you just go into any sporting goods store and pick up a tennis racket that seems to fit your hand.

If you have an identified predisposition to joint problems, avoid any sports that may promote degenerative changes, and seek out other, less risky physical workouts. J. A. Buckwalter of the Department of Orthopaedic Surgery at the University of Iowa Hospital points out that people with anatomical defects or early osteoarthritis can benefit from regular physical activity, "but they should have a careful evaluation of their joint structure and function before participation. They should consider measures that decrease the intensity and frequency of impact and torsional loading of joints, including use of sports equipment that decreases joint impact loading, maintaining, or improving muscle strength, tone, and general condition so that muscle contractions help protect joints from injury and high impact, and decreasing body weight."

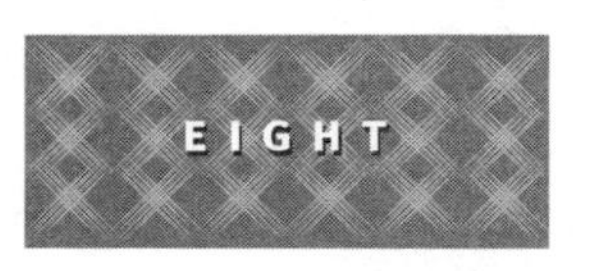

Eat Right and Take a Load off Your Joints

Early in my career I treated a patient named Mabel, and the image of her is still fresh in my mind. She was about forty-six when I first saw her. She stood five-foot-four at the most, and weighed about 345 pounds. I treated her for various ailments, including pain in her knees. Over the next several years, the pain grew worse. Then she complained of pain in the ankles. By the time she was fifty, her knees were in very bad shape. She became more and more immobile and eventually wheelchair bound. I remember her husband rolling her, jammed into a wheelchair, into the office. I also remember trying unsuccessfully to convince her to lose weight.

When I started practicing medicine, it was thought that excess weight could contribute to osteoarthritis, particularly of the knees. In medical school, I had heard my professors allude to the connection between weight and arthritis. But there was no emphasis on it. Our training focused merely on what to give patients for relief of pain when they developed arthritis. And in the hospitals in those days, dietitians were more concerned about keeping patients happy than addressing a food-related weight problem.

As a young doctor, I began to see the overweight-arthritis connection among my patients. Many of them were extremely heavy. I was making about twenty-five house calls a week and became aware of how overweight individuals with arthritis quickly became immobile. In so many houses I visited, I would see an overweight arthritic patient sitting on the couch, feet propped up, watching TV on one of those early black-and-white sets, and munching on a plate of snacks.

The more immobile they were, the worse the arthritis became. And the heavier they became. After a time, it became quite evident that these heavier people were not living as long as thinner patients. I soon realized that unless I could inspire them into activity and working on their weight problem, the disease process would be relentless and irreversible.

Nearly a half-century later, two things have become very clear:

1. Excess weight raises the risk of developing osteoarthritis.

2. Losing weight lowers the risk.

David T. Felson, M.D., the Boston University expert on osteoarthritis, has estimated that weight reduction could substantially cut the risk of symptomatic knee and hip arthritis. In one of his studies, conducted over a twelve-year period, women who lost just eleven pounds decreased their odds of developing knee arthritis by more than 50 percent. Although there is little data per se on weight loss as a treatment for osteoarthritis, "the preliminary information suggests it is especially effective in knee disease and that even small amounts of weight reduction may have favorable effects," says Felson.

The challenge is how to lose the weight if you are too heavy.

How to Tell If You Are Overweight

The government has developed a simple guideline. It's called the Body Mass Index (BMI).

Basically, the BMI is your weight in kilograms (2.2 pounds = 1 kilogram) divided by height in meters (39 inches = 1 meter) squared.

If you don't want to do the math, some Internet websites

have simple forms where you type in your weight in pounds and height in inches, click on the submit button, and get your BMI level. That's a whole lot easier. You will find, for example, a BMI calculator at *www.drkoop.com/tools/calculator/bmi.asp.*

Experts agree that the "ideal" BMI scores should range from 19 to 25. Overweight is considered 25 to 29.9, and over 30 is obese. A person five-foot-nine and weighing 180 pounds has a BMI of 26.5, while at six-foot-one with the same weight the BMI would be 23.7. Someone five-foot-three and 150 pounds has a BMI of 26.5. But at five-foot-seven and 150, the BMI is 23.4.

the missing link in weight loss

In 1959, I began sharing a medical practice with Murray Medoff, M.D. My speciality was in pain, his was in treating excessively overweight patients. It was Medoff who coined the term *bariatrics* to describe this medical specialty. He shared many of his research findings and clinical experiences with me and contributed considerably to my understanding of weight reduction. It gave him great joy to see a patient lose weight and keep it off. And in my own practice, I felt similarly gratified to see a patient with chronic pain lose enough weight to relieve the problem.

In those days, amphetamines, amphetamine-like drugs, and huge amounts of thyroid medication were commonly used to obtain weight loss. These substances were potent weight reducers and metabolic stimulants, but they frequently generated side effects such as tremors and anxiety. Their use worked for the short term, but patients wouldn't continue taking them for long. Moreover, the body became adapted to the medication, and higher doses were needed. I saw patients lose considerable weight, but then they would gain it back again because the body was no longer responding to the medication.

In time I came to regard any drug approach to weight loss—for most people—as a sure failure and potential danger. Recent events certainly bear this out. In 1997 the Food and Drug Administration called for the withdrawal of the popular appetite suppressant Fen-Phen because of increased incidence among female users of valvular heart disease. In 2000, a Yale University study linked PPA (phenylpropanolamine), an ingredient in many cold medicines and diet pills, to an increased risk of deadly stroke in women under fifty. An advisory panel of the FDA declared that the chemical should no longer be considered safe.

Los Angeles, where I have practiced medicine for many years, is the mecca of thinness obsession. As a medical "weight watcher" for decades, I have consistently observed thousands of patients enthusiastically start some fad diet and then soon quit and go on to something else. I came to the conclusion years ago that weight-loss diets don't work. Statistics say that 98 percent of weight control programs fail, and I can't argue with that figure. Most patients won't stay on a diet program for any significant length of time. The programs are too complex or restricting for them.

I have also observed that weight-loss programs, even those prescribed by weight-loss specialists, are generally doomed to failure unless they are accompanied by an exercise program. For this reason, I always emphasize exercise to all my patients who need to lose weight. This has been my weight-loss gospel for years. In my experience, it's not just the calorie intake, but the calorie expenditure as well.

To date, unfortunately, physical activity has not been emphasized in most treatment programs for overweight and obesity. Yet inactivity, as we have seen, is an independent predictor of premature death. Obesity experts are now calling for more public awareness of the importance of balancing energy intake with physical activity.

New research has emerged over the last decade proving that physical activity is a critical factor contributing to successful body-weight regulation. In a review published in an international journal on obesity,

W. H. Saris of Holland's University of Maastricht pointed out that "individuals who are successful in long-term maintenance of weight reduction are highly likely to be physically active. Participation in physical activity is among the best predictors of success in weight maintenance. Physical activity facilitates weight maintenance through direct energy expenditure and improved physical fitness."

Steve Blair, P.E.D., of the Cooper Institute in Dallas, has studied the role of exercise on health for two decades. His findings include these two important points:

- Regular physical activity clearly minimizes many of the health risks associated with overweight or obesity.
- The addition of exercise to diet programs produces more weight loss than does dieting alone and is especially important in maintaining weight loss in overweight persons.

In advising patients as to how to lose weight, I felt I needed to keep the recommendations as simple, and yet as effective, as possible. My approach to diet became very pragmatic as well. I recommended a calories-in, calories-out approach that meshed exercise and diet. You took in a certain amount of calories; you used up a certain amount of calories in your daily activities, which included exercise.

I found that most of my heavier arthritic patients could significantly reduce their symptoms if they followed—and maintained—a good diet and exercise program. I also observed that for the most part, those patients who maintained a normal weight had fewer arthritic problems in the weight-bearing joints. I sensed that if they did develop arthritis in those joints, it manifested later than with heavier patients.

I always recommend slow and steady weight loss, not the big-numbers approach of some pop diets. People who lose weight rapidly tend to put it back on as fast. People who lose it slowly tend to keep it off.

At this point I would like to share my calories-in, calories-out (CICO) program with you. I am also including some other principles I have learned over the years in regard to eating that may help you in your attempt to eat well, feel well, and keep your weight at a healthy level.

calories-in, calories out (the CICO diet)

The CICO formula can work wonders for you in a relatively short period of time if you follow its three-part approach:

- the vitamin C cocktail
- simple calorie counting and good nutrition
- daily exercise (or five times a week) for at least thirty minutes

CICO Part 1. The Vitamin C Cocktail

One of the major challenges of trying to lose weight is to eat less, a much more palatable wording than "suppressing appetite." Any plan involving suppression of appetite is doomed from the start in my opinion. Moreover, medications that suppress the appetite can be dangerous to use for long periods of time, or else they lose their effectiveness fairly fast. Hunger and appetite are natural expressions of health in every living creature. Food is the fuel of energy, cell growth and repair, and the countless biochemical processes consistently in motion within our bodies.

Vitamin C can help you eat less.

Here's the concept: You take vitamin C a half-hour before meals. It helps reduce the feeling of hunger by creating a counterfeeling of fullness in the stomach, as well as a sense of hunger satisfaction, or satiety. Your pangs of hunger can thus be relieved even before you take a bite.

In addition to this unique benefit, vitamin C is an extremely healthful substance. Among its many contributions to the body, it is a potent antioxidant, protecting tissues from harmful oxidative effects that lead to disease and accelerated aging. It protects the immune system, the entire heart and vascular system, promotes wound healing, helps rid the body of toxins, and is a major component in tissue integrity, including the collagen so vital to joint cartilage. Vitamin C also is a natural painkiller. And in case you have a problem with sweets, it cuts the craving.

The vitamin C cocktail is made simply by dissolving a rounded teaspoon of vitamin C crystals (about 5 grams) in 16 ounces of water (1 pint).

That's enough for two meals. You will be drinking 8 ounces of the fluid each time.

The form of vitamin C crystals that I prefer is sodium ascorbate. It is buffered, that is, it has a neutral pH and is not as tart as the more common ascorbic acid form of vitamin C. There is no problem using ascorbic acid crystals if you don't mind the taste.

Many health food stores have vitamin C in the crystal form, usually as ascorbic acid. In some cases you may have to special order it, and particularly so if you want sodium ascorbate. You can also order the crystals from major distributors such as Bronson Pharmaceuticals (800-235-3200). Most economical is to order a pound or even a kilo at a time.

Prepare the cocktail in advance and keep it in a cool place until you need it. The liquid is fairly stable and can be prepared twenty-four to forty-eight hours in advance. If you wish to make a full quart at a time, then use two teaspoons of the vitamin.

Shake the mixture well, not only at the time you make it, but also just before you use it. There is no problem if you wish to use any flavoring such as condensed lemon juice or fresh lemon or lime juice. Don't use anything with sugar since that would add calories to the drink. Nor do I recommend any fructose, since calories are eventually absorbed from fructose and add to your daily caloric load, which you are trying to keep down.

During the many years I have recommended this practice, I have not found any patients who have suffered any dangerous or severe side effects that warranted discontinuing the vitamin. Some patients found that the 2,500 millgrams (2.5 grams) of the vitamin before a meal caused a slight, temporary diarrhea. They then reduced the dosage and had no more problem. Most people can use vitamin C in this way. If you are under the care of a physician, ask your doctor about doing this. Be sure you are not one of those few people who are allergic to vitamin C.

CICO Part 2. The Diet

Divide your daily diet roughly into 40 percent protein, 30 percent carbohydrate, and 30 percent fats. To determine the number of calories you need daily, proceed as follows:

1. Select your ideal weight.

This can be determined by asking your physician or utilizing a simple formula used by many doctors:

- For women, 100 pounds for the first 5 feet, and 5 pounds for each additional inch.
- For men, 106 pounds for the first 5 feet, and 6 pounds for each additional inch.
- If you have a large frame, add 10 percent; if a small frame, subtract 10 percent.

For the sake of an example, we will use the figure 154 pounds as an ideal weight.

2. Figure your weight in kilograms.

To do that, divide your weight by 2.2 pounds (one kilogram). The kilogram weight in our example is 70.

3. Figure your ideal caloric intake.

To do this, multiply your weight in kilograms by 24 (hours in the day). For 70 kilograms, the amount would be 1,680 calories.

4. Adjust your calories according to your activity level.

Are you sedentary or active? Factor in your exercise and working activity to determine your adjusted caloric intake level. If you are a basically sedentary person, allow yourself an additional 20 percent calories. Allow 30 percent if your activity is light, 40 percent if moderate, and 50 percent if vigorous.

Let's illustrate this step by using our example of 70 kilograms. If you do light exercise (such as walking for 30 minutes a day), multiply 1680 by .30. That would give you an extra allowance of 404 calories for a total of 2,084. This then would be the number of calories you need to maintain 154 pounds and exercise or work at a light level or activity.

5. Figure your percentage of protein, carbohydrates, and fats.

Take the calorie total from step four and divide it into the percentages of protein, carbohydrates, and fat. In our example, 2,084 calories are equal to about 833 calories of protein, 625 of carbohydrates, and 625 of fats.

6. Don't lose too much too fast.

A reasonable, healthy goal is 1 to 2 pounds a week. To do this, reduce your ideal caloric intake total (from step 4) by 500 calories if you want to lose 1 pound a week. Reduce your intake by up to 1,000 calories a day to lose 2 pounds. Do not under any circumstances lower your daily intake below 1,200 calories.

7. Choose your food.

So much has been written about the best food for weight loss. I don't want to add to the mountains of confusion that already exist. However, a good diet maximizes fresh, wholesome food and minimizes the amount of nutrient-depleted processed food.

8. General points

- *On protein.* In our society there is no end of opportunities for eating protein. A three-ounce piece of red meat every day or two is fine and not going to cause any problems. Eggs are great. I like to see patients eat more fish, and particularly salmon. I value the benefits of fish, with its good protein and high content of omega-3 fatty acids, for cardiovascular health and also for the joints.

  The wide variety of soy products offers strict vegetarians good alternatives for animal protein.

- *On carbohydrates.* Your body breaks down carbohydrates and sweets into glucose, also called blood sugar. This is the basic fuel used by cells to perform their specialized functions. Unless you provide a steady supply, you can develop muscle weakness and a whole variety of physiological problems.

  The body controls the sugar level and entry into the cells with insulin. When the sugar level in the body rises too high, more insulin is produced, driving the blood sugar level down. After a meal of too many carbohydrates or sweets, your energy can drop precipitously to a state of fatigue, depression, or irritability. Such blood sugar fluctuation is called hypoglycemia, and the degree of change necessary to produce symptoms varies from person to person.

  A condition called hyperinsulinemia can develop from constant overproduction of insulin. This, in turn, can be a forerunner to major metabolic disturbances, including insulin resistance and diabetes. Interference with cellular operations occurs. Cells lose their ability to receive and process information delivered by insulin and other hormones.

  Elevated insulin also causes problems with fat processing in the body and results in increased fat storage and weight gain. If you suspect any insulin problem, consult with your physician.

  Mounting scientific research indicates we process dietary carbohydrates into body fat more readily than the fat we eat. The problem in our society is that we eat far too many carbohydrates: pretzels, chips, bagels, cookies, cake, pasta, bread, rice, and potatoes. The more carbohydrates you eat, the more insulin produced by the body, and the more fat storage that occurs.

Be careful with your intake. Eat about one-third of your total calories as quality complex carbohydrates (such as whole grains and vegetables). Avoid sweets as much as possible. If you have a sweet tooth, I recommend a wonderful Indian herb called *Gymnema sylvester* to help cut your craving. You'll find it in health-food stores. Take a standardized extract twice a day.

- *On fats.* You must learn to stop looking at fats as your enemy. Fats are necessary to maintain life. In fact, many hormones, including estrogen, progesterone, and testosterone, are derived from fats. The vital lining around many nerves, as well as the membranes of cells, are fatty substances.

Too little fat in the diet, or eating only one type of fat, is a ticket for potential trouble. You need a variety of fats.

Try to increase the amount of omega-3 fats in your diet because we eat too many of the omega-6 types of fats, those found in meat and polyunsaturated cooking oils. I talk more about this important dietary issue, and how it relates to joint health, in the next chapter. Refer to the section on omega-3 fatty acids.

There are certain fats that are not healthy for you. As much as possible, stay away from fried foods and hydrogenated and partially hydrogenated fats, found in many processed and baked goods.

Reduce the amount of saturated fats in your diet. That includes butter, lard, and animal fats. Don't replace butter with margarine, as that is not a healthy type of fat. Just use butter sparingly.

If you favor low-fat food, beware of what you are buying. Some of the highly palatable low-fat foods contain added sugars and other ingredients that render the foods high in calories. Using such products as substitutes for fattier foods is likely to bring about only small reductions in calorie intake. A better strategy to reduce calories is to eat more fruits, vegetables, and other foods high in fiber and complex carbohydrates.

CICO Part 3. Exercise

I have covered exercise in depth in chapter 7. It has been proven over and over that exercise is one of the most effective ways to take off weight. This is especially true if your caloric load is held steady or reduced to the basic calorie needs of your body.

For effective weight loss, aim for moderate exercise thirty to forty-five minutes five times a week.

Exercise builds up muscle, and muscles operate at a higher metabolic rate. This means you burn more calories.

It's also a fact that exercise raises your overall metabolic rate. For a few hours after exercise your body is also burning additional calories.

it's not just what you eat but how you eat!

Don't gobble your food. Fletcherize, or chew very slowly while you eat. Don't be in a hurry. Take time to masticate. Cultivate a cheerful appetite while you eat. So will the demon indigestion be encompassed . . . and his slaughter complete.

—JOHN D. ROCKEFELLER *NEW YORK EVENING MAIL*, 15 MAY 1913

Today, in an age where eating on the run has become a standard way of eating, the fundamental act of mastication suffers badly. People seem too busy to chew their food adequately and may even be getting lazier about it, suggests Susan Schiffman, Ph.D., professor of medical psychology at Duke University.

"Why do people like ground-up hamburger meat?" she asks. "Because they don't have to chew it as much. There's less effort. I think that people who don't chew enough swallow larger bites and have more stomach trouble and take more antacids."

Proper chewing is essential to health and, by the way, a terrific and totally overlooked avenue to weight loss. That was a lesson dramatized by a health enthusiast named Horace Fletcher a hundred years ago. He was probably the greatest crusader for chewing in the history of the world.

Fletcher had been a "gulp-eater" like most of us are today. We have grown accustomed to gulping down our food as we read, watch TV, or talk throughout meals and to giving scant attention to chewing our food.

Fletcher was forced to pay attention to chewing because his life was on the line. Before the turn of the last century, he was a fortyish college professor—extremely overweight, beset with poor health, chronic indigestion, and limited energy. During a trip to Europe to restore his vitality he came across a statement made by former English prime minister William Gladstone that bites of food should be chewed thirty-two times, or once for each tooth.

That made sense to Fletcher, so he tried it. And he tried other things related to how you eat, such as never eating when you are tired, disturbed, or angry; never eating until you are hungry; and keeping away unpleasant thoughts at mealtime.

Applying these principles, Fletcher regained his health within a half-year, totally conquering fatigue and illness. He lost fifty pounds. With newfound vigor he entered long-distance bicycle races and even outperformed college athletes in feats of strength and endurance. He also wrote and lectured widely on his eating style, which became known as Fletcherism. Among his followers were leading physicians, politicians, and the Rockefellers.

Chewing Your Way to Health

Horace Fletcher promoted his eating style through physical feats, often performed with much hoopla and publicity at the Yale University gymnasium.

In 1907, at the age of fifty-eight, he claimed a world record of sorts by lifting 300 pounds of deadweight some 350 times with the muscles of his right lower leg on an endurance-testing machine developed by Yale professor Irving Fisher. The previous record had been 175 lifts.

Later that same year, he lifted 770 pounds with the muscles of his back and legs, "a feat that weight-lifting athletes find hard to perform," he wrote in his 1913 book, *Fletcherism: What It Is, or, How I Became Young at Sixty.*

"I performed these stunts eating two meals a day, one at noon and the other at 6 P.M., at an average cost of eleven cents a day," he said.

On chewing, Fletcher went beyond Gladstone's suggestion and recommended fifty chews per mouthful. He told people to count while they chew, to chew their food to a pulp until it practically swallowed itself, and to face downward so the food could slip easily through the "food gate" at the back of the mouth.

Fletcher's ideas may seem extreme, but he made people think about chewing. Indeed, chewing is the first step in digestion. Properly done, it breaks food down into smaller, more digestible pieces while at the same time mixing the food with saliva. The saliva contains enzymes that begin the digestive process, particularly for carbohydrates and starches, and it lubricates the food for a smooth drop down into the stomach.

As the chewing starts, the stomach begins to produce its own lubricating and breakdown juices that further enhance the digestive process.

Most people can't resist swallowing or talking for the fifty chews recommended by Fletcher, but maybe for the sake of digestive efficiency and weight loss we should aim to chew more and gulp less.

your eating environment

Rarely, it seems, do people sit down just to eat. They usually sit down to eat and talk, eat and read, or eat and watch TV.

"People talk too much and chew too little," says Duke's Schiffman. "Talking between chewing would be a better habit. It would slow you down."

Slowing down in fact may be a valid strategy for losing weight. As head of a weight-loss clinic at Duke, Schiffman has learned from her patients that wolfing down food with hardly a break between bites results in excessive amounts of food in the stomach. By contrast, slow, careful chewing seems to put less food in the stomach. More time is spent on chewing and less on swallowing, giving the person more of an opportunity to get in touch with feelings of fullness.

Additionally, the more you chew, the more you taste. Chewing forces air—and odor—back into the nose through your throat.

"That's the way we get most of our odor and taste from the food we eat," says Schiffman. "We don't smell it through the nostrils. We get it retronasally. When you put it into your mouth you may think it is taste, but it is really odor that is going up the back of the throat and being picked up by the nose."

It is perhaps for the gustatorial benefits of chewing that hard-core epicureans would agree that the meal table is a place to conduct the business of eating rather than business while eating. "Conversation is the enemy of good food," was the way the late, great movie director and gourmet Alfred Hitchcock once put it.

However, eating is more than a nutritional activity. It is also social.

So eating in monastic silence isn't always appropriate, but you get the idea. Mealtime may be a good time to listen and let others do the talking. If you need to lose weight it's something to consider.

keeping your digestive "fire" hot

Some of the oldest dietary recommendations in the world come from India's Ayurvedic medical tradition, some five thousand years old. There are two central considerations in the Ayurvedic approach to diet. One is *agni,* a Sanskrit term meaning "digestive fire," or, as we understand it in the West, the mechanisms and enzymes involved in digestion. The other main element is *ama,* the impurities produced by poor digestion and metabolism.

D. Edwards Smith, M.D., a board-certified rheumatologist, internist, and expert in Ayurveda, says a strong *agni* yields good health through efficient digestion and metabolism that breaks down food properly, makes its nutritional components available to the tissues, and removes waste products and toxins from the body.

"*Ama,* on the other hand, is 'sticky' by nature, and basically adheres to tissue that is somehow anatomically disrupted," he points out. "If you have channels in the body that become plugged, the tissue that is 'downstream' becomes inflamed, shrinks, or becomes deformed. Channels in the body come in all shapes and sizes. They include the gut, the blood vessels, the lymphatic system, and even the gaps between cells and molecules.

"If you have any kind of injury or trauma, that means anatomical disruption. The ancient Ayurvedic texts described injuries such as falling off elephants and fast-moving chariots. That's not likely to occur in our day but the opportunity for trauma is nevertheless present anywhere and in any age. And if you have a lot of *ama* in your body, it tends to stick in these places of disruption or previous injury, and the sites are often the joints."

While we have some but not total control over preventing injuries, we can do much to prevent the accumulation of *ama,* says Smith, dean of the Maharishi College of Vedic Medicine in Albuquerque. First and foremost is eating according to the laws of nature. That means the following:

- If possible, eat at the same time every day. Follow the natural digestive rhythms. Ayurveda says to eat the largest meal at lunch, when digestion is strongest. Dinner should be a modest meal that can be digested before bedtime.
- Do not eat until you are hungry. Snacking between meals interferes with the process of digestion and creates *ama*. Allow three to six hours between meals.
- Sit down when you eat. After each meal try to remain seated and quiet for a few minutes instead of jumping up and rushing into activity. That enables your body to better switch into digestive gear.
- Preoccupation with talking, reading, or watching TV while eating disconnects your awareness of how much is being eaten as well as the sights, smells, tastes, and textures of the food. This sensory information is vital to the brain and facilitates the complex process of digestion by the stomach and intestines. Extraneous mealtime activities contribute to overeating and overweight.
- Digestive ability is diminished if you are ill or under much stress. Eat lighter.
- Eat your food hot or at least warm.
- Avoid cold drinks, and particularly ice drinks, with meals. It is recommended to sip hot water instead. Cold beverages extinguish *agni* and thus promote *ama*. Hot water improves digestion and appears to help keep open the countless channels throughout the body. In

ancient Ayurvedic times, there was no ice cream. Because of its coldness, Ayurvedic physicians discourage ice cream at the end of a meal.

- Eat food that is as fresh and chemical free as possible.
- Food that is easiest to digest is best for you. This means that well-cooked food is preferred over raw and hot over cold.
- "An excellent diet can be planned around foods that the timeless Ayurveda tradition has found most beneficial," says Smith. "However, there are no blanket prescriptions so it is best to have professional guidance in selecting the diet best for you." Diets are prescribed by Ayurvedic physicians according to specific body types and imbalances. Ayurveda recognizes biological differences among individuals and creates preventive and therapeutic programs based on these differences. Body types are determined according to size, structure, skin, hair, color, pulse, tastes, habits, temperament, and preferences. Such diets, along with specific herbs, detoxification, massage, meditation programs, and sound therapies, are tailored to individuals by Ayurvedic physicians to promote ideal health.

The CICO Diet has worked for a lot of my patients. But it is still a diet. You just may not be a diet person. If you think it is more than you want to follow, or honestly think you can't do it, then the simple approaches of Ayurveda may work for you. Apply as many of them as you can in the pursuit of good digestion and weight loss.

The main thing to remember is to eat to the point of satisfaction, not of fullness. That means about three-quarters of your capacity. One way to do this is to cut down on desserts and fried foods. Most people won't cut them out, but cutting down can make a difference.

The late Wilt Chamberlain, who played professional volleyball into his fifties after his great basketball career ended, was once asked by a reporter how he kept the weight down on his huge frame. "I push myself away from the table," he answered.

Chamberlain would probably have agreed with Maimonides, the illustrious Spanish physician of the twelfth century, who said that "most maladies afflicting humanity result from bad food or an excess of food that may even have been wholesome."

So, from ancient times to the present, eating less is a golden rule. And it has particular relevance for our overeating society.

Try also not to eat within six hours of bedtime. Drinking fluids is OK, preferably water. If six hours isn't practical because you may not eat until seven or eight o'clock after returning home from work, try for three or four. The idea is to burn off the calories of the last meal before you go to sleep. When you sleep and still have a big meal in your digestive tract, the contents are more readily converted to fat than if you were to burn off the calories with activity.

Most Americans eat their largest meal late in the day. I see that as a major problem contributing to our overweight epidemic. Eating late, or giving in to the infamous midnight snack urge, are to be avoided.

I encourage my patients to eat their biggest meal at lunchtime, which follows the Ayurvedic understanding that digestion is strongest at midday. This is a difficult habit to develop because the act of eating has so many social aspects to it, many of which are related to dinner. One of the benefits of eating dinner early is that you awake good and hungry, which is as it should be.

Many Americans skip breakfast, and miss the meal that provides "takeoff" fuel for the day's activities. As a result, hunger develops at midmorning and you grab whatever is handy from the vending machine, office kitchen, or mobile caterer, and it is usually food low in freshness, wholesomeness, and nutrient value. Some people don't eat until lunch, at which time the hunger may promote overeating.

One more thing about eating: Do make an effort to include plenty of fresh fruits and green leafy vegetables in your diet, and, if possible, make your food choices organic. Americans tend to come up short on these very important foods. You are what you eat, so why settle for anything but the best and most nutritious food you can buy?

the fiber-obesity connection

Between your mouth and your rectum is a fifteen-foot-long tube—your digestive system. Food enters, gets chewed up, torn to shreds by enzymes, acids, and bacteria, and, when all goes well, is absorbed into the bloodstream. The unused and undigested parts are expelled at the far end of the system—the colon, also known as the large intestine.

In physiological terms, transit time refers to the time it takes for food to get through this biological maze. In a healthy body, thirty hours should do it. That's common in primitive societies where people eat a natural diet. Here, however, in our constipation-prone society, forty-eight hours and more is the norm. This means the end products of digestion remain in our system longer and become smaller and harder to expel. In time, the colon becomes a waste dump for toxins, harmful bacteria, and carcinogens, a breeding ground for disease and malfunction.

A leading guarantor of good transit-time intestinal health is dietary fiber, also known as roughage. Fiber is the portion of plant food that human digestive enzymes cannot break down. It is most readily available in *complex* carbohydrates—*whole* grains, *whole* grain pasta, seeds, nuts, natural fruits, beans, and vegetables. Fiber absorbs moisture, increases in size, gives the muscles in the intestinal walls something to grip, makes the stool softer, and acts as a natural laxative.

Research shows you have a higher risk of developing major infirmities of the colon, including cancer, as well as cardiovascular disease, if you don't eat enough fiber.

Fiber also plays an important role in calorie intake control and thus serves in the interest of arthritis prevention. Here is how a diet rich in fiber helps keep weight down:

- Fiber has unique physical and chemical properties that enhance the sensation of satiety.
- Fiber lowers insulin. The more insulin produced by the body, the more fat storage occurs. High insulin is also associated with increased free-radical damage, a leading contributor to disease.

Researchers think that fiber consumption may be an even more important factor in preventing obesity and cardiovascular disease than lowering fat consumption. This was the conclusion reached in one study at the Children's Hospital in Boston where nearly three thousand healthy young adults have been monitored for more than ten years.

Unfortunately, here in America and other industrialized countries, we fail to eat enough vegetables, fruits, and *whole* grains. In short, not enough fiber. Instead, we overeat fast, fiberless, fat-filled, fabricated food.

We also fail to drink enough water (see chapter 10) and get enough exercise (see chapter 7). The lack of these fundamental elements in daily life creates constipation and the backup of toxins in the body, and it affects all of the physiology and anatomy, including the joints.

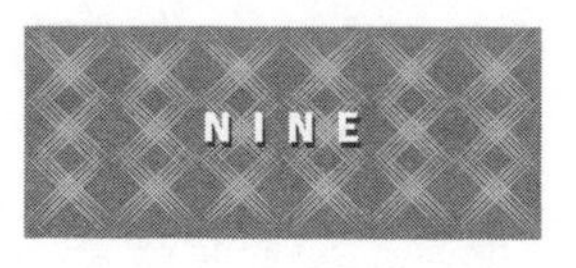

Supplement Your Joints

The way we eat in America—unbalanced diets typically heavy in processed, devitalized foods—can impact health in a big way. Nutritional surveys conducted periodically by the U.S. Department of Agriculture consistently show huge numbers of Americans with low or suboptimal intakes of essential nutrients such as calcium, iron, zinc, magnesium, and vitamins A, B1, B2, B6, and C. The scientific evidence links these low intakes to the risk of serious health consequences.

How do such deficiencies occur in the land of plenty? Here's how:

- Two-thirds of the food we eat is processed, depleting vitamin and mineral content.
- Sugar and highly processed refined carbohydrates comprise an estimated 60 percent of the average American diet. These are "empty calorie" foods—poor in nutrition, high in fat—that force your body to "borrow" nutrient reserves to digest the junk.
- Intensive farming and long-term use of chemical fertilizers and pesticides have caused the serious loss of nutrient content in agricultural crops.
- Canning, cooking, storage, freezing, and preparation cause major nutrient loss.
- Fast food, the symbol of the modern American diet, is notoriously deficient in vitamin A, several of the B vitamins, iron, and copper.

- Oral contraceptives, used by an estimated 10 to 18 million American women, deplete vitamins B2, B6, B12, C, E, folic acid, and zinc.
- Alcohol destroys the vitamin B complex group and vitamins A and C, along with zinc, magnesium, and calcium.
- Aspirin, perhaps the least toxic of painkillers, speeds up the urinary loss of calcium, potassium, the B vitamins, and vitamin C.
- Chemical and emotional stress increase the body's need for certain vitamins.
- More than three thousand chemicals are used in commercial food. Many of them can affect nutritional status.

These facts help explain in part why chronic illness is rampant in the United States and they also make a strong case for nutritional supplementation. Clearly, we should all eat as well as we can. That should be the priority. And then on a solid foundation of wholesome food, we should optimize our nutritional intake with supplements.

An explosion of research on nutrition and nutritional supplements has taken place during the last ten years. Many studies now prove that individual nutrients at doses higher than those usually present in the diet can have a profound preventive and therapeutic impact against serious diseases. Massive consumer interest and a torrent of scientific discoveries about vitamin, mineral, amino acid, herbal and so-called nutraceutical supplements have also prompted increased usage among physicians.

Can supplements work to prevent wear-and-tear arthritis, which has so many possible risk factors, including age, gender, weight, trauma, and joint overuse?

Unfortunately, the wonder supplement has not been sighted yet that can neutralize each and every risk factor and keep arthritis at bay. But researchers and clinicians are showing how supplements can exert significant therapeutic benefits such as slowing down disease progression and minimizing symptoms. We also think that some supplements, by themselves or in combination, may delay the onset of osteoarthritis and help protect the joints. This is a dynamic field that should continue producing exciting news in the years ahead.

In this chapter, you will find a comprehensive review of a powerful array of supplements with joint-protective benefits. And in order to help you use them in an effective way, I have combined them at the end of the chapter into an arthritis prevention supplement program.

A Short Guide to Buying Supplements

Avoid "bargain" prices.

Cheap products usually mean cheap ingredients and contents that may be below the potency claim on the label.

Stay with quality, reputable brand names.

vitamin C

Vitamin C does so much in the body. You definitely don't want to be caught short.

Vitamin C is a big player in joint health, where it serves as a biochemical partner in the production of collagen, the connective tissue in cartilage that holds the proteoglycans in place. Specifically, collagen contains sizable quantities of an amino acid called 4-hydroxyproline. Vitamin C is needed to facilitate the enzymatic processing of a precursor amino acid, proline, into 4-hydroxyproline for the production of collagen.

Researchers have repeatedly demonstrated how important vitamin C is to healthy cartilage. Laboratory experiments have shown that chondrocyte cells isolated from bovine cartilage and cultured with vitamin C produce a more extensive matrix rich in collagen and proteoglycans. Human skin cells cultured with vitamin C also produce more collagen.

In the early 1980s, researchers at Tufts University School of Medicine took laboratory experimentation one step further by seeking to determine the role of vitamin C supplementation in animals. They used guinea pigs, who, like humans and monkeys, do not produce their own vitamin C. The vitamin must be obtained in the diet.

The researchers supplemented the guinea pigs with either minimal or maximal amounts of vitamin C to analyze the effect on arthritic joints. The findings showed that animals on minimal levels of vitamin C "always" exhibited more pathology than those on high levels. As the disease progressed, there was consistently more pitting, ulceration, and overall thinning and degeneration of cartilage. Cartilage weight in normal joints was greater for the animals kept on a high dose of the vitamin. The researchers commented that the higher level likely stimulated production of cartilage and protected the animals against the severe deterioration found in the minimally supplemented guinea pigs.

In human medicine, Frederick Klenner, M.D., of Reidsville, North Carolina, was a leading pioneer in the therapeutic use of vitamin C. During decades of clinical practice, he used quite large doses and published many reports in medical journals. In one report he said flatly that "a person who will take 10–20 grams of ascorbic acid (vitamin C) a day along with other nutrients might very well never develop arthritis."

While that may seem like a huge amount of vitamin C, it was the kind of dosage that vitamin C champions like Klenner, Linus Pauling, and other nutritionally oriented experts have advocated for the treatment of a wide variety of conditions. "Repair of collagenous tissue is dependent on adequate ascorbic acid," said Klenner, who also pointed out that taking regular high doses of aspirin or cortisone to ease arthritic pain depletes vitamin C in the body.

Vitamin C has other qualities that make it a very joint-friendly nutrient. For instance, it is a potent free-radical scavenger. Free radicals, as you will remember from chapter 2, are molecular substances produced in the body that are involved in many degenerative disease processes and accelerated aging. Researchers have found that free radicals are produced in cartilage tissue by the chondrocytes and believe that this activity may contribute to degeneration.

At Boston University's Arthritis Center, Timothy E. McAlindon, M.D., and colleagues published a statistical study in 1996 reporting significantly less disease progression among people with osteoarthritis of the knees who had a higher dietary (food and supplement) intake of vitamin C. In the study, individuals averaging from 150 to 500 milligrams daily had a third of the progression of those whose intake was below 100 milligrams. A higher level of vitamin C appeared to be "protective against cartilage loss," slowing down progression and reducing the risk of developing knee pain, the researchers reported.

Their study failed to find a significant connection to the incidence of knee osteoarthritis. Antioxidants such as vitamin C, they said, could have a greater role in "preventing progression rather than incidence," which can result from a variety of risk factors such as knee injury, repeated stress from occupational activities, and obesity. They called for further investigation.

Over the years, my patients who took good doses of vitamin C seemed to display less symptoms of connective tissue disorders, including osteoarthritis. While many patients had X ray indication of arthritis, and even quite advanced cases, they appeared to have less pain. Vitamin C also has a reputation as a pain reliever. Early in my practice I used to give it intravenously on a weekly basis to many arthritic patients as a significant adjunct to pain relief treatment.

How Much Vitamin C to Take

- Minimum of 500 milligrams daily

vitamin D

Degenerative change in the bone tissue—called subchondral tissue—just beneath the cartilage spells trouble for the joint. Such change can cause a loss of shock absorption, stability, and repair capacity. Metabolism in this tissue and throughout the bones requires vitamin D. When the vitamin is in low supply, researchers think that the support from bone tissue to counteract arthritic processes is compromised.

At the Boston University's Arthritis Center, researchers also found that individuals with a higher dietary intake of vitamin D had a third less progression of knee arthritis than those with low intake. Low D was associated with loss of cartilage and the development of osteophytes.

In a different study, researchers found that high levels were protective against both the incidence and progression of hip arthritis.

How Vitamin D Much to Take

- 400 international units (IUs) daily

You may not need to take this much in a supplement if you are routinely exposed to sunlight. Sunlight converts a precursor to vitamin D in the skin. However, you may not be able to obtain the sunshine benefit during the winter months in the northern part of the country.

People over fifty have less ability to produce the vitamin precursor in the skin and may need up to 600 IUs daily. Those over seventy may need 800 IUs.

Cod liver oil or fatty fish are good natural sources of vitamin D.

vitamin E

Moti Tiku, M.D., associate professor of medicine at the Robert Wood Johnson Medical School in New Brunswick, New Jersey, is a leading investigator of free-radical activity in cartilage tissue.

Researchers know that the chondrocytes—the cells that produce the proteoglycan and collagen molecules in cartilage tissue—also produce many free radicals, but they don't know yet the purpose of this activity.

More than ten years ago, Tiku and his research colleagues started developing sophisticated laboratory methods that would allow them to study these molecular goings-on within cartilage tissue.

"We wanted to see whether the collagen matrix is broken down because we know that such breakdown would be a critical step in the development of osteoarthritis," says Tiku.

Experiments in his laboratory and elsewhere have demonstrated that indeed the chondrocytes produce certain free radicals that break down the fatty components in their own membranes and also create damage in the surrounding collagen matrix.

"This may possibly be a factor in osteoarthritis," says Tiku, "but the research is really in its infancy and we don't know yet if the free radical activity in the matrix is playing a major or minor role in the degradation of cartilage in our joints."

In his most recent experiment, Tiku found that the degradation could be almost entirely prevented by the addition of vitamin E to the chondrocyte cell cultures. Vitamin E is a well-known antioxidant nutrient that inhibits the free-radical activity that is present, for instance, in the formation of arterial plaque and the aging process.

Tiku's experiment raises the question as to whether vitamin E also has a protective role specifically in osteoarthritis.

He thinks it holds the promise. "I believe we can make a logical inference from our research that vitamin E may offer preventive benefits," says Tiku.

No other studies have been conducted testing whether vitamin C or coenzyme Q10, other known antioxidants, have similar effects. "I am sure they will be done," he adds.

This exciting line of sophisticated scientific investigation has opened a fascinating avenue for prevention possibilities. However, it will take more research like this to determine definitively whether antioxidant supplementation offers significant protection not just in the laboratory but in our bodies.

The direct effect of vitamin E on patients with osteoarthritis was first reported in the sixties. Newer studies, particularly in Europe, indicate that the vitamin reduces pain and allows patients to use less medication.

How Much Vitamin E to Take

- 400 international units (IUs) daily of natural vitamin E (d-alpha tocopherol)

glucosamine and chondroitin sulfate

Until the bestseller *The Arthritis Cure* (St. Martin's Press, 1997) introduced glucosamine and chondroitin sulfate, most people in the United States had never heard of them. Now they are practically household words, and are widely sold as nutritional supplements.

Glucosamine is a major constituent of connective tissue, including cartilage. Made in the body from glucose and the amino acid glutamine, it is used by chondrocytes to make proteoglycans, the molecules in cartilage that hold water. Chondroitin is the most abundant glucosaminoglycan (GAG) in the body. GAGs are the sugar units attached to proteins that form proteoglycans.

Glucosamine supplements are derived from the shells of crabs, lobsters, and shrimp. Chondroitin sulfate is prepared from bovine (including calf) cartilage.

In Europe, glucosamine and chondroitin have been used therapeutically (they are prescription items) and researched for thirty years. In one major European study, announced at the 1999 annual conference of the American College of Rheumatology, researchers found that glucosamine not only significantly reduced pain and improved movement for patients with arthritis of the knee but also prevented joint-space narrowing. During this study, conducted over three years, researchers at the University of Liège in Belgium compared 139 patients, some of whom took 1,500 milligrams of the supplement daily, and others of whom took an inert placebo.

Joint-space narrowing is an indicator of the degenerative process. The term refers to the thinning of cartilage tissue. The process of narrowing is usually quite slow, and thus requires an extended period of time to analyze.

At the start of the Belgium study, and again after one year and three years, the researchers took standard X rays of the patients' knees. When the X rays were analyzed, the patients receiving a placebo were found to have an average joint *narrowing* of .31 millimeters (about a hundredth of an inch). This represents a typical loss of cartilage for someone with osteoarthritis. A slight but statistically insignificant increase in joint space was noticed in the glucosamine group. Symptoms worsened among the placebo takers, but not among the glucosamine users.

Another important element to this study was that it showed for the first time relief of symptoms over several years, an advance over previous research that generally lasted only a few months. Many American experts who had previously criticized glucosamine trials as being too short in duration hailed this study. None of the prescription anti-inflammatory drugs, by the way, have undergone a study of such length, according to Jason Theodosakis, M.D., the lead author of *The Arthritis Cure*. A second, confirmatory study of similar design was presented at the 2000 meeting of the American College of Rheumatology.

Glucosamine supplements are available in two forms—sulfate or hydrochloride. Both are beneficial. Some supplement companies have claimed that the glucosamine sulfate form is more effective, but such claims do not stand up to scientific scrutiny. In fact, when you take a glucosamine sulfate supplement, it is converted to the hydrochloride form by stomach acid. The only head-to-head study published so far revealed that glucosamine hydrochloride had a slightly greater ability to stimulate production of the cartilage-building proteoglycans.

New European studies with chondroitin, involving both animals and humans, show this natural agent also helps improve the joint space in the hips, knees, and fingers. One three-year double-blind study at Ghent University Hospital in Belgium examined the impact of chondroitin on osteoarthritis of the fingers. Chondroitin or a placebo was given to 119 patients. At the end of the study, the researchers concluded that chondroitin protected against "erosive evolution" of the joints.

The ability of both glucosamine and chondroitin to deter such structural damage in the joints has earned them the reputation as chondroprotective agents, that is, substances that protect cartilage.

These supplements are widely used by consumers, health professionals in the alternative medicine community, and an increasing number of rheumatolgoists. In general, the medical community is looking ahead to a major four-year study in the United States that was launched in 2000. Both glucosamine and chondroitin sulfate are being tested in this study, which will be funded by the National Institutes of Health and involve more than a thousand patients.

Many patients have asked me which of the two—glucosamine or chondroitin—is more effective. To answer that question I asked *The Arthritis Cure*'s Theodosakis, who has been using these supplements routinely in his medical practice since the early 1990s and closely follows research developments.

"Both the research and my own personal experience with patients demonstrate that glucosamine shouldn't be used alone," the Tucson physician points out. "I have seen a lower rate of improvement and frequent 'rebound' of symptoms among patients who took only glucosamine. I would estimate that only about 60 percent of patients improve if they take glucosamine alone, a figure that is similar to research findings. The research indicates clearly that chondroitin has a much greater therapeutic impact than glucosamine.

"In a March 2000 report published in the *Journal of the American Medical Association,* experts reviewed all of the double-blinded, placebo-controlled studies of glucosamine (six such studies) and chondroitin (nine) performed before July 1999. Analyzing the studies yielded the conclusion that the clinical treatment effect of chondroitin almost doubles that of glucosamine. Chondroitin is much more important than glucosamine. This finding matches my own clinical observation that chondroitin is well absorbed and acts much longer in the body."

These revelations were surprising to me because glucosamine has received far and away more media attention. I have also heard claims made by some marketers of glucosamine that chondroitin is not well absorbed; however, such claims are not supported by the research and are vehemently rejected by Theodosakis.

"Any assertions of this nature are untrue, as well as a grave injustice to individuals suffering from osteoarthritis," he says. "Chondroitin is certainly absorbed. None of the placebo-controlled studies would have been positive if this were not so. In addition, the effect of chondroitin lasts for months."

Even though Theodosakis regards chondroitin as the more powerful compound of the two, he does not recommend it alone. "I always recommend taking both. They work synergistically, and you get better results. A new and important animal study has shown that the combination is dramatically more effective in minimizing cartilage damage. A large human study is under way to confirm this."

Users can expect the following results from the combination, according to Theodosakis's clinical experience:

- Decreased pain
- Increased range of motion
- Ability of arthritic patients to do more physically
- Ability of arthritic patients to reduce their reliance on pain pills
- Reduced swelling, and a lessening of the "cracking" noise that is sometimes heard from affected joints.

Theodosakis says about 80 percent of people with arthritis who take the combination experience these results. The degree of improvement is individual, he points out, though; improvement may occur at any age and even in cases where X rays show severe bone-on-bone joint deterioration.

I also asked Theodosakis how glucosamine and chondroitin rate as antiarthritis agents compared with standard NSAID medications.

He told me that studies have shown that these two natural substances are as effective as NSAIDs in relieving pain: "They have anti-inflammatory effects, like NSAIDs, but they do much more than just relieve pain. Unlike NSAIDs, which decrease cartilage formation, glucosamine and chondroitin stimulate the formation of new cartilage tissue. And because of that they take longer to achieve maximum effect. There is evidence that the longer the supplements are used, the greater the benefits. Four to five months is really the minimum to try them."

Moreover, unlike NSAIDs, there have been no reports of serious side effects with glucosamine and chondroitin, Theodosakis says. "Conventional medications used for osteoarthritis can cause peptic ulcer, liver damage, or kidney disease. This does not happen with glucosamine or chondroitin. Nor do they have any interactions with drugs, including NSAIDs and acetaminophen, so the supplements can be taken with medication if necessary.

"Keep in mind that glucosamine and chondroitin are not simply pain medication and don't act immediately like painkillers. Still, some people notice pain relief within the first few days. My advice is to be patient, because the results can be very rewarding."

If you try glucosamine and chondroitin and notice only a marginal effect in pain relief, Theodosakis recommends, you should still consider using the supplements long term. "It is important to think of them not only for pain relief but for their cartilage-protective effects, to help prevent or slow down further deterioration," he says. "Cartilage loss and pain are often not connected. NSAIDs and acetaminophen reduce pain, but the cartilage continues to deteriorate. Glucosamine and chondroitin enhance cartilage repair and have a secondary effect at reducing pain."

In a purely preventive approach, Theodosakis feels strongly that glucosamine and chondroitin can be beneficial to individuals with risk factors for osteoarthritis who have not developed symptoms. That includes younger people who may be constantly traumatizing their joints through sports activities. He also recommends the supplements for people who have had joint surgery for cartilage tears or fractures that affect joint cartilage.

buyer beware!

If you are ready to run to the health food store or visit your favorite Internet vitamin supplier to order the glucosamine/chondroitin combo on sale, hold your horses. *There's a major caveat here.*

After the publication of his bestselling book, patients began reporting to Theodosakis that they were not getting results from many of the glucosamine/chondroitin supplements combinations they bought through various outlets.

"They would complain that the supplement worked only temporarily," he says. "I began to suspect that some of the products didn't have the actual content that the labels claimed. In particular, I thought there might be little or no chondroitin in them, since chondroitin is very expensive to produce and is the most important component of the combination. Supplement potency for chondroitin is crucial."

To determine if his suspicions were correct, Theodosakis began sending products to an independent laboratory and paying for an analysis out of his own pocket. "These were the products, many of them popular brands, on which I had the most reported failures," says the doctor. "Sure enough, the lab results corresponded to the failures. Companies were skimping on chondroitin, and sometimes massively."

In one test he conducted in 1998 of one hundred three samples, 78 percent had a level of chondroitin short of the label claim. Some also were below label claim in glucosamine. "Some products contained less than 5 percent of what they claimed on their label. The testing of one major brand shocked me. It had 1.1 percent of the label claim in thirteen out of fourteen lot samples tested. Instead of the claimed 400 milligrams of chondroitin in the capsule, it had 4.4 percent. No wonder patients were telling me consistently that it didn't work. When they switched to a brand I recommended, they got results."

Because it was his book that first brought the benefits of glucosamine and chondroitin to the attention of the American public, Theodosakis is angered by supplement marketers who sell deficient products. "If this is done intentionally, it is outright fraud. If it is not intentional, there is still no excuse. It's the business of companies making and distributing these products to know."

I asked Theodosakis which commercially sold combinations he feels comfortable recommending. Although he has not tested every product on the market, as of February 2001 he said the following brands met or exceeded label claims, based on analyses of multiple lots:

- Osteo Bi-Flex Glucosamine Chondroitin (Manufacturer: Sundown)

- MaxiLife Glucosamine & Chondroitin Sulfate (Twin Labs)
- Gluco-Pro 900 Glucosamine Chondroitin (Thompson)

Theodosakis's testing program is ongoing. For more information about what's up to par, and what is not, visit his website at *www.drtheo.com*

How Much Glucosamine and Chondroitin to Take

- Glucosamine: a daily total of 1,500 milligrams, usually in one or two doses
- Chondroitin sulfate: a daily total of 1,200 milligrams, usually in one or two doses

MSM

After the 1999 publication of *The Miracle of MSM: The Natural Solution for Pain* (Putnam), the use of MSM has soared. The book, which I coauthored with Stanley W. Jacob, M.D., and Martin Zucker, brought attention to a very remarkable supplement supplying the body with sulfur, an overlooked mineral that is a major component of protein compounds. Sulfur contributes to countless biochemical and structural activities, and is a stabilizing element in cartilage, tendons, and ligaments.

MSM (as noted earlier, short for methylsulfonylmethane), is a biologically active form of sulfur and offers powerful benefits that make it a favorite among arthritic patients and individuals with chronic pain conditions. Here is what MSM does:

- It reduces pain by inhibiting pain impulses that run along nerve fibers.

- It acts as an anti-inflammatory.
- It decreases muscle spasm around arthritic joints, which also helps relieve pain.
- It lessens the formation of scar tissue.
- It improves blood flow throughout the body.
- It may slow down the degeneration of cartilage.

Over many decades, medical studies have indicated that sulfur levels in arthritic joints are lower than normal. In a 1995 study, the concentration of sulfur in the arthritic cartilage of horses was shown to be about one-third the level of normal cartilage. This figure was comparable to sulfur measurements reported during the 1930s when physicians used intravenous and intramuscular injections of sulfur for arthritis.

Sulfur has a long healing tradition. Throughout history, healers and physicians have sent ailing patients, and particularly arthritics, to soak in sulfur-rich hot springs.

MSM supplementation often provides significant improvement—less pain, less stiffness, and greater mobility—for people with osteoarthritis, and even for severe cases. Within two to four weeks, and sometimes sooner, patients commonly start feeling better. I have often been able to reduce the dosage and sometimes even eliminate the use of strong painkillers as a result, and other physicians have told me the same thing.

In some very severe cases, MSM may postpone the need for hip or knee replacement. Replacement techniques are improving all the time. So if MSM can postpone surgery by even a year or two, the potential for a more successful outcome is enhanced.

Laboratory and clinical experience suggest that MSM slows down joint deterioration associated with arthritis. At Oregon Health Sciences University, studies were conducted during the 1980s with rodents known to spontaneously develop a joint disease similar to rheumatoid arthritis. When some of the animals were supplemented with MSM they developed significantly less cartilage deterioration than animals who were not supplemented. Such research involved rheumatoid arthritis, and not osteoarthritis, but experience with patients points toward a delaying or protective effect for osteoarthritis as well.

Preliminary research that I have been conducting suggests a chondroprotective effect of continuous supplementation with 3,000 milligrams of MSM daily. This positive indication is based on MRI studies of the knees, and lumbar and cervical spine, of osteoarthritis patients who have been taking MSM for a year. The images taken at one year showed no evidence of joint-space narrowing when compared to pictures taken at the start of the study. This is a sign that the process of deterioration may have been arrested. The imaging study is still in progress.

an amazing letter

As coauthor of *The Miracle of MSM,* I have received numerous letters from readers who experienced such great relief that they were inspired to sit down and tell their stories. No letter amazed me more than the one from Robert Ansley, Jr., a forty-six-year-old roofing and sheet-metal contractor from Shallotte, North Carolina. He wrote me a seven-page, single-spaced letter six months after starting a combined MSM-glucosamine combination. The effects, he said, were "astounding, dramatic, nearly immediate, almost overwhelming, and to me, nearly miraculous."

Ansley suffered from severe osteoarthritis and calcification in his back and knees, as a result of years of hard physical labor in construction, farming, and truck driving. His feet and an elbow were painful to him as well. He had also had many injuries, both minor and major, along the way. He said he spent a fortune on doctors and painkillers.

"There were so many times and instances of being bedridden, walking with a cane and all kinds of braces, that they all blend into a blur in my memory," he wrote. "Despite it all I was young and strong enough to slog through it and slough it off. But time and age and the accumulation of injury conspired against me. Increasingly, I was unable to push on. Until July 1999, I was always hurting somewhere. If it wasn't my back, it was my knees. If not my knees, it was my neck, shoulders, or elbow. And, oh yes, my feet and lower legs hurt all the time. I really thought my productive life was over."

In July 1999, Ansley started taking MSM and glucosamine.

"It hit me in just over twenty-four hours after the first dose," he wrote. "There was an increase in energy like I had never experienced before. My elbow, which was extremely painful at the time, stopped hurting. I was flabbergasted."

Ansley said that during the following week he was astounded to realize that his feet and legs didn't hurt, and then his back and knees stopped hurting.

"Everything stopped hurting," he said.

It's been nearly a year and half since Bob Ansley started taking MSM and glucosamine.

"I never hurt anymore," he reported in the fall of 2000. "The only pains I have now are from occasional injuries. I haven't taken any kind of painkiller for nearly a year. The worst thing I've had to do is rub some MSM on a twisted wrist or overworked knee and those things are rare now. All of the energy I have is being well used getting back into life. I come home legitimately tired and sleep like a baby most of the time."

Ansley said he took very high amounts of MSM. He found that it took 36 to 40 grams (36,000 to 40,000 milligrams) "to get rid of all my chronic pain."

This is much, much higher than people should take on their own without a physician's supervision. I only advise patients to take high amounts when they are open to it and when I am able to monitor them closely.

In Ansley's case, he stayed at the peak level for almost half a year and then began to notice dryness in his nasal passages and eyes. He also developed a small mouth ulcer. Sensing that these might be mild side effects from too much MSM, he stopped taking the supplement for three days and the symptoms disappeared. He subsequently found that 30 grams of MSM is what it took to give him the relief he desires without any discomfort.

In his personal experimentation to find the most effective combination of dosages for him, Ansley determined that higher levels of MSM and not of glucosamine produced profound results. He reported additional healing of his back problems by adding hydrolyzed collagen (HCP), Ester-C, and an amino acid combination, and working closely with a skilled chiropractor.

This suffering North Carolina man's story may not be typical. Not everybody gets results, and so dramatic, and so fast. But most people do experience some degree of improvement, some fast, some slow. The letters from readers of our book indicate that MSM offers a safe form of relief, in combination or by itself. There is nothing to lose by trying it and, as Ansley wrote, possibly a whole new painfree life to gain. Remember that we are all individual. Some people will respond at lower doses, others at higher doses. If you have any doubts about what is safe for you to take, consult with your physician. From my experience, MSM is very safe. Just watch for any signs of discomfort, an indication that you have exceeded your individual tolerance. If you overdo it, you may develop minor gastrointestinal discomfort, more frequent stools, or a mild skin rash. Just reduce the dosage if that happens. With this or any supplement or medication, you always want to take the least amount necessary to give you relief.

Currently, MSM is also found as part of joint-health formulas along with ingredients such as glucosamine and chondroitin sulfate. Patients have often said they obtain better results by using these multiple ingredient formulas. These formulas vary widely in their contents and it is not possible to offer an opinion on which combinations are better than others. They may have an advantage in that there is a synergistic effect from combining multiple substances. There is, of course, a practical benefit from a formula supplement. You don't have to take as many pills.

If a particular combination works, fine. If it doesn't, you may want to try another, or refer to my suggested combinations of joint-related supplements you can put together yourself.

How Much MSM to Take

- For maintenance and general health, take 3,000 milligrams or less each day. Patients with osteoarthritis and other pain problems often use 3,000 to 8,000 milligrams.

Take the supplement with meals.

Many of my patients, including actor James Coburn, have experienced remarkable relief from severe arthritis problems with MSM, and prefer taking the supplement in the crystal (powder) form. They simply mix the crystals into water or juice. If you have difficulty finding MSM crystals in your favorite health-food store or pharmacy, you might like to try the quality product I recommend to my patients: Mega MSM, distributed by GeroVita International (800-586-4649; or on the Internet at *www.gvi.com*).

For musculoskeletal problems such as osteoarthritis, I also recommend applying an MSM lotion or gel to the affected area. MSM penetrates the skin, carrying anti-inflammatory and pain-killing properties into the area of the affected joint. If you cannot find a lotion at a nearby store, contact MSM manufacturer Carolwood Corp of Greenville, Pennsylvania (phone: 888-646-0350; or on the Internet at *www.msm.com*), or such major distributors as Natrol (800-326-1520; *www.natrol.com*), Natural Balance (800-833-8737; *www.naturalbalance.com*), Jarrow (800-726-0886; *www.jarrow.com*), or Now (800-999-8069; *www.nowfoods.com*). Another good option for topical relief is an effective spray containing MSM, glucosamine, menthol, eucalyptus oil, and peppermint oil. Called Stop Pain, the product is marketed by DRJ Group in Carlsbad, California (800-801-7246).

Higher amounts of MSM may be necessary to experience therapeutic effects for very severe, chronic arthritis. Always start low. Increase your dosage slowly. Many people start off with 2 or 3 grams a day and increase another gram or two after several days. As you raise the level of MSM, divide the doses during the day. Take the MSM with meals. If you encounter any discomfort in your intestinal tract, or a mild skin rash, reduce the amount you are taking. When such signs disappear, slowly raise the amount again. If you develop the same discomfort, your body is saying that's the limit. Although many people take high amounts of MSM without any problem, some individuals are unable to take more than just a small dose.

MSM does not interfere with medication.

B complex vitamins

Some of the B complex vitamins that have shown considerable promise against osteoarthritis in the past have been largely forgotten today. They shouldn't be. I strongly recommend B complex vitamins to my patients. Not only do they have powerful protective benefits for the nervous and cardiovascular systems, but also for joint health as well. B complex factors are present in multivitamin formulas. For therapeutic effects, as detailed in the information below, you will need higher doses.

Niacinamide

Niacinamide is a form of vitamin B3. You may be more familiar with the other form called niacin, often prescribed to lower cholesterol. But niacin can also cause an uncomfortable flush of the skin that feels like an allergic reaction. Niacinamide does not create the flush.

In the 1940s, a Connecticut physician named William Kaufman, M.D., found that niacinamide could significantly improve arthritis symptoms and he prescribed this nutrient with great success for many thousands of patients over five decades.

Kaufman's discovery was that many arthritis patients were dependent on vitamin B3. They often needed a large dose of the nutrient, far exceeding the amount occurring in the diet. Today's recommended daily allowance (RDA) is 19 milligrams for men and 15 milligrams for women. However, most nutritionally oriented physicians view the RDAs as far short of optimum levels and even further short of the therapeutic benefits that specific nutrients offer at high, safe dosages.

In Kaufman's case, he found that 500 milligrams of niacinamide four times a day was a very safe and effective dosage. The reason it needed to be taken so often was that the vitamin is rapidly excreted. Frequent supplementation ensures an effective blood level.

In 1955, Kaufman reported his findings to the *Journal of the American Geriatrics Society*. He described his experience based on 663 patients in his private practice who took niacinamide (alone, or in combination with other vitamins) for periods ranging from a few months to nine years.

Without exception, individuals who took 900 to 4,000 milligrams of niacinamide in divided doses each day had clinically significant and measurable improvement in joint mobility, regardless of age, according to Kaufman.

Many patients, especially older individuals, noticed a significant improvement in strength and exercise tolerance soon after starting the program. This effect reached a peak during the first three months and continued as long as the vitamin was continued. Improvement occurred within three months or would not occur afterward with niacinamide alone. However, when B1 (27 milligrams) and B2 (54 milligrams) were added to niacinamide, some patients experienced rapid improvement in muscle function. Some needed choline, another B complex vitamin, in the amount of 2.4 grams taken in divided doses, before they experienced improvement in muscle function.

"Surprisingly," Kaufman reported, "in patients with weak, flabby muscles who benefited from choline . . . there was development of muscle resilience and tone to a degree expected in people who do moderately heavy physical work—even though these patients continued their sedentary existence." Kaufman believed that choline supplies methyl groups, substances needed for the enzymatic and metabolic processes that give rise to muscle power.

For individuals whose muscle function was below par, the vitamin program raised their level to normal. Lower normal levels were raised to upper normal. Niacinamide and the other vitamins raised patients "to a state of vigor which permitted them to perform duties without excessive fatigue, whereas they had been unable to do so before treatment," he said.

Niacinamide, either alone or in combination with B1, B6 (54 milligrams), and B12 (twice a week injections of 100 milligrams), significantly improved balance and the sense of steadiness and muscular coordination of many older patients.

Niacinamide has a beneficial effect on nervous-system function. Kaufman found it helped many older patients with mild chronic depression. Some patients also required additional B1, B6, and B12 for relief from depression.

No patient experienced any negative reaction to niacinamide at any time. Improvement was maintained for as long as patients took the vitamins.

Kaufman's experience suggests that the addition of a B complex vitamin supports niacinamide and provides further benefits.

In an age when clinicians were first applying new discoveries in vitamin usage, Kaufman found that his approach could "reconstitute" some of the functions of the aging body. Here was a true pioneer, someone way ahead of his time. It wasn't until a half-century later that his consistent findings inspired a modern-day study. It was conducted by W. B. Jonas, M.D., and colleagues, at the National Institutes of Health's Office of Alternative Medicine and reported in a 1996 issue of the journal *Inflammation Research*.

In this carefully controlled double-blind study, sixty osteoarthritis patients at a small community hospital completed the trial in which they took either niacinamide or an identical-looking placebo pill on a daily basis for twelve weeks. The patients were all over forty years of age, symptomatic for at least five years, and had joint pain and X ray evidence of arthritis in at least two joints.

Participants received one 500-milligram tablet of niacinamide six times a day—a total of 3,000 milligrams. They continued their regular arthritis medication for pain and adjusted the level as needed during the study.

Jonas's group confirmed that niacinamide "improved the global impact of osteoarthritis, improved joint flexibility, reduced inflammation, and allowed for the reduction in standard anti-inflammatory medications."

Beneficial effects were felt within one to three months. Even better results occurred later among those who continued using the supplement for one to three years.

The dosage level used in the study appears to be safe, according to the study. Forty percent of the niacinamide users reported mild GI responses such as gas or loose stools, which were controlled by taking the vitamin with food or fluids.

The researchers suggested that megadoses of niacinamide increase the levels of certain elemental substances in cartilage and synovial fluid. This, in turn, provides the energy and raw materials important for cartilage repair in the deeper layers of the cartilage matrix. The effect could "increase cartilage repair rates," they believe.

Abram Hoffer, M.D., Ph.D., a Victoria, British Columbia, specialist in nutritional medicine, has found that niacinamide can substantially reduce pain and improve impaired range of motion due to arthritis.

"I first observed the benefits of niacinamide on arthritis patients in 1953, and have continued to see good responses ever since," he says. "Many physicians have also told me over the years how arthritic symptoms improve with the vitamin."

Hoffer believes that "if niacinamide had been a patented drug, there is little doubt it would be one of the main treatments for arthritis today."

Adds Melvyn R. Werbach, M.D., a leading medical researcher and author of *The Textbook of Nutritional Medicine* (Tarzana, Calif.: Third Line Press, 1999), "unfortunately, when he passed away in August of 2000, Kaufman had not received the recognition he deserved for his pioneering arthritis work, nor has it been thoroughly followed up as one would expect. He documented the benefits of niacinamide for a huge number of clinical cases, helping people with many different degrees of arthritis. He thoroughly quantified their illness before and after treatment."

How Much Nicinamide to Take

- Preventively: as part of a B complex or multivitamin formula
- Therapeutically: 500 milligrams three or four times a day

vitamin B6

John M. Ellis, M.D., a self-declared "country doctor serving the local folks," forged ideas in his practice over decades that have impacted the lives of people far beyond the cattle and bass country of northeast Texas where he lives. In thousands of cases, the Mt. Pleasant physician found a vitamin B6 deficiency involved in arthritis, as well as carpal tunnel syndrome, the edema of pregnancy, complications of diabetes, and cardiovascular disease. When he corrected the deficiency with B6 supplementation, he was often able to clear up or improve many signs and symptoms of illness.

Ellis is probably the world's leading champion of B6. He has presented his clinical findings to physicians and researchers at international medical forums and passionately carried his message of supplementation to Native American tribes, where the incidence of diabetes is exceptionally high.

Ellis, now eighty-four and retired, zealously practices what he preaches. He has taken B6 regularly for nearly forty years.

"I don't have a bit of arthritis," he says proudly in his Texas drawl. "I can stand on one foot and put the other foot up on the kitchen table with my arms extended out to the side and hold my balance for a long time."

Vitamin B6 deficiency is fairly widespread. According to a recent National Health and Nutrition Examination Survey conducted by the U.S. government, the average daily intake of B6 is 2.07 milligrams for men and 1.47 for women. The recommended daily allowance (RDA) is 2.2 milligrams for men and 2 milligrams for women. Bananas, avocado, and other raw fruits and vegetables are primary sources of B6.

"But people don't eat enough of these foods," says Ellis, who recommends 100 to 200 milligrams daily.

B6, and other B complex vitamins, are depleted in the highly processed foods that are overconsumed in the United States. Alcohol and excessive protein, fat and sugar intake rob the body of B6. Cooking, boiling, and baking eliminate up to 40 percent of the vitamin. Women taking oral contraceptives have been found to have a B6 deficiency. The level of B6 also declines significantly in older age.

This is no small matter, because, as Ellis says, "there are 118 known enzymes that are dependent on B6 to perform essential functions in tissue and blood chemistry," among them regulation of hormones, metabolism of proteins and carbohydrates, and proper function of nerve cells.

The exact biochemistry of how B6 helps arthritis is not clearly understood. However, researchers have shown there is a close relationship between the biological activity of the vitamin and the regulation of the major steroid hormones, including estrogen and progesterone in women, and testosterone in men, as well as cortisol.

"Cortisol may be the big one," says Ellis. "Cortisol is an anti-inflammatory substance. B6 regulates cortisol and helps to move it in and out of tissues."

B6 also has a property that enables it to pull excess fluids, such as occur with edema, out of tissues. Ellis believes that part of the vitamin's pain-relief benefit comes from generating positive changes, such as removing excess fluid from the elastic tissue of the joint capsule.

According to Ellis, there are sixteen signs and symptoms indicative of a B6 deficiency. The most important include numbness and tingling of the hands, impaired sensation in the fingers, morning stiffness of finger joints, pain in the hands, thumb joint, shoulders, and elbows, and tenderness over the carpal tunnel (wrist area).

"People will first notice numbness and tingling in the hands and fingers," he says. "Other signs develop gradually and become more severe as time goes on. They don't all appear at first, but they appear later on as severity increases. Low-grade, sub-clinical discomfort can go on for years and then you may develop the real arthritic symptoms of stiffness and pain around joints. This is particularly the case with women, in my experience."

Ellis believes that an unrecognized B6 deficiency may be involved in arthritic symptoms occurring with aging.

"When B6 is taken preventively, there are simply less symptoms, and not just relating to arthritis," he says. "Taking 100 milligrams daily can prevent an A to Z of problems. Prevention is in the picture because I have seen so many patients who have improved signs and symptoms after starting on B6. If they would have taken it years before, I believe they never would have developed the problems. That's because B6 does so much in the body."

During his nearly four decades of medical practice, Ellis honed B6 therapy into a fine art. He treated thousands of patients, including many with osteoarthritis.

"In my experience I have seen a frequent association of pain in the hands, elbows, shoulders and knees that respond very well to a B6 program," he says. "The recommended dosage is the same—100 to 200 milligrams daily."

Ellis recommends starting at 100 milligrams and then evaluating the situation after three months.

"Usually there is improvement, but if signs and symptoms persist, go up to 200 milligrams, and evaluate yourself again after two or three months," he says. "The pain and stiffness in the knees beginning in middle age will usually respond to 100 milligrams of B6 daily. You will first notice the pain decreasing, and then the stiffness eases up, and you will be able to walk and get around better."

Other painful joints should respond similarly. And among women, a stiffness in the fingers known as Heberden's nodes responds specifically to B6. In this condition, spurs develop in the finger joints, causing unsightly bumps, stiffness, and pain.

"Here once again, 100 to 200 milligrams helps relieve the pain, improve the flexibility of the joints, and remove a bit of the redness," Ellis says. "The vitamin can make a significant difference for women who can't write because they can't flex their fingers. B6 won't remove the spurs. Nothing will do that. You try to prevent them."

How long does it take to see results with B6?

"It normally takes four to five weeks of daily use to adequately enhance dependent enzymes and maximize their function," he says. "Then it takes another four to five weeks to get a reversal of signs and symptoms of deficiency. A total of about three months."

The Texas doctor points out that the vitamin is much more likely to work better in the early stages of arthritis and may be much less effective for very severe cases.

How Much Vitamin B6 to Take

- Preventively: 100 milligrams daily
- Therapeutically: 100 to 200 milligrams

omega-3 fatty acids

Omega-3s are an important group of fatty acids you have probably heard about in connection with cardiovascular health. These natural substances help thin the blood, reduce high blood pressure, decrease triglycerides, and cut down inflammation in blood-vessel linings and joints.

I began recommending omega-3 fatty acid supplements in the form of fish oils more than ten years ago for their cardiovascular benefits. But I soon found that patients with osteoarthritis benefited as well. I believe this has to do with the effect of omega-3s on inflammation.

In osteoarthritis, the calcium deposits that frequently develop press or rub like sandpaper against the synovial lining, resulting in inflammation and pain.

Omega-3s have yet to be proven clearly beneficial for osteoarthritis. The studies just haven't been done. But according to Artemis P. Simopoulos, M.D., president of the Center for Genetics, Nutrition, and Health in Washington D.C, and a world authority on fatty acids, the evidence points to a protective and therapeutic role.

"We know that we need to raise our dietary intake of omega-3s," says Simopoulos, author of *The Omega Diet* (HarperCollins, 1999). "That's because of a huge increase in recent decades in the use of omega-6 foods, primarily vegetable cooking oils, that has caused an alarming imbalance.

"Bones consists of two major types of cells—osteoblasts and osteoclasts," she explains. "Osteoclasts break down bone tissue, which is then resorbed. Osteoblasts create new bone tissue. This is a continuous process that maintains the proper metabolic condition of your bones."

Prostaglandin E2 is a hormonelike substance, derived from an omega-6 fatty acid called arachidonic acid, and it increases the production of osteoclasts. You need adequate vitamin E and omega-3s in the diet to reduce this activity and restore balance. (The terms omega-3 and omega-6 refer to the particular chemical structures of fatty-acid molecules.)

The dietary imbalance relates to a food supply with an increasing use of cooking vegetable oils (such as corn, safflower, and sunflower) high in omega-6 fatty acids compared to omega-3s. Corn oil, for instance, has a ratio of 60 to 1. Safflower has 77 to 1. Adding to the imbalance is the typically high intake of meat, eggs, and dairy products, all containing much more omega-6s than 3s. Experts say that the overall ratio of omega-6s to -3s in today's Western diet ranges from between 20 to 1 and 30 to 1, compared with an evolutionary ration of 1 or 2 to 1.

"This is a type of diet we shouldn't be eating," says Simopoulos.

The omega-3 fatty acids are primarily EPA (eicosapentaenoic acid) and DHA (docosahexaenoic acid) found in fish oils, and ALA (alpha-linolenic acid) found in flaxseeds, soybeans, walnuts, and green leafy vegetables. In the body, ALA is broken down into EPA and DHA.

"On the basis of animal studies, researchers are suggesting that too much omega-6s in the diet and not enough omega-3 fatty acids contributes to accelerated degeneration of the bone," Simopoulos says. "In experiments, EPA and vitamin E seems to counteract the effect of arachidonic acid.

"Unfortunately there are no controlled human clinical trials on osteoarthritis and omega-3s to date," she adds. "But we can make the point that bone is the supporting foundation of cartilage, and in order to maintain normal bone metabolism, you appear to need adequate amounts of omega-3 fatty acids and vitamin E to offset the omega-6s. We have very little of the omega-3s in our diet, and too much omega-6. Too much of the 6s interfere with the balance of the metabolism.

"The animal research and what we know about normal bone metabolism tells us it is wise to balance the 3s and 6s in your diet. You want to promote normal bone metabolism and decrease the risk for fractures. This risk is increased among people with osteoarthritis because there is some loss of balance that goes along with the condition. With bones becoming more brittle and more prone to fracture with age, keeping bones strong is very important for older people, both women and men."

Simopoulos also points out that in research involving elite athletes, inflammation and pain can be reduced with high amounts of the antioxidants vitamin E and co-enzyme Q10, along with EPA. The research has indicated that rheumatoid arthritis patients who have very little omega-3s and high amounts of interleukin-1 (an inflammatory substance found in the plasma and in the joint fluid of rheumatoid patients) can be helped with supplementation of omega-3s.

"The studies strongly suggest that supplementation with omega-3 fatty acids counteracts the effects of the omega-6," she says. "Supplementation can bring down the inflammation and people feel better."

In recent laboratory studies in England using cartilage cell cultures, researchers have found that the introduction of omega-3 fatty acids can reduce the activity of the damaging and inflammatory compounds that cause cartilage destruction in arthritis. The findings, said the Cardiff University investigators, further support the evidence of a beneficial role for supplementation.

In April 1999, Simopoulos participated in a National Institutes of Health workshop that recommended supplementation of about 650 to 1,000 milligrams of EPA and DHA daily. These are the omega-3 fatty acids derived from fish oils. Alternatively, the workshop suggested, adults can use 2 to 3 grams of alpha-linolenic acid daily, such as is available in walnuts, canola oil, flaxseed, and flaxseed oil. By the way, dark green leafy vegetables are a good source of alpha-linolenic acid as well. Some fifteen years ago Simopoulos headed a group of researchers who discovered that purslane, a plant once used widely as food and medicine by Native Americans but ignored today, is the richest source of omega-3s among vegetables.

In my practice I have used higher amounts of omega-3s with excellent results. I have recommended capsules containing 1,000 milligrams of fish oil, of which about 300 is EPA or DHA. Some patients take as many as sixteen capsules a day. On average, they take between six and nine, equaling 1,800 to 2,700 milligrams of the omega-3 fatty acides.

Personally, I burp or "repeat" after taking fish oil supplements. I have found that about two out of ten patients experience a similar sensation. That's why I was glad to learn about an alternative called perilla oil, an Asian plant with a long history of medicinal and cooking use. Perilla is rich in omega-3s. In fact it contains more than fish oil. If you experience discomfort from fish oil you may want to consider Entrox, a quality perilla supplement that is enteric coated for maximum absorption. It is made by Carolwood Corporation of Greenville, Pennsylvania (phone: 866-4ENTROX). Perilla is also known as Chinese basil or purple mint. It has been widely studied in the Orient.

Another burp-reducing option is Coromega, a fish oil supplement made by ERBL of Carlsbad, California (phone: 877-275-3725). It contains orange flavoring, making it more palatable, and comes in unique packaging that allows you to squeeze the daily dose into your mouth or onto a spoon or food.

Simopoulos says that the higher dosages of omega-3 supplements that have been widely used are not generally necessary if the amount of cooking oils and other omega-6s are lowered in the diet.

"The idea is to decrease the intake of omega-6 and increase omega-3, and when you do that, you only need to increase the omega 3s moderately," she says. "This is the approach for both prevention and treatment, although for treatment you may need to increase the amount."

I certainly agree with this. Reducing omega-6s is important. Nevertheless, I have a few dozen patients still taking six to nine capsules a day and doing very well. I just saw one of them, a sixty-eight-year-old male patient, who has been on nine capsules a day for ten years. He is in great shape. No heart problems. No joint pain.

Another patient is a fifty-year-old waiter and active surfer. He looks thirty-five. He was taking MSM and was very much helped for pain in his right knee. But he still had persistent pain. He added three capsules of fish oils a day. Two weeks later he reported back and said the pain was gone.

Hopefully, says Simopoulos, we will obtain more definitive answers on the use and benefits of omega-3s when the proper studies are done. The need for such studies, she adds, has attracted the attention of the government "and once the government becomes interested, there will be studies."

How Much Omega-3 Fatty Acids to Take

- Preventively: Follow label instructions.
- Therapeutically: 2 to 3 grams.

boron

When he was forty-five years old, Australian soil scientist Rex E. Newnham developed osteoarthritis in the feet and knees, which made walking increasingly painful. His prescription medication failed to help him, so he set out to find what was causing the arthritis. His investigation led him to suspect that the fruits and vegetables he was eating were deficient in boron, a mineral needed by plants for proper calcium metabolism.

Newnham decided to try ingesting a bit of boron and see if that helped him. Not only did it help him, but within a month his pain and stiffness were gone. He told other people with arthritis about his experience. They too tried boron, and over time, hundreds reported similar results. His boron revelation, almost forty years ago, inspired a lifelong crusade to promote the use of boron as a nutritional aid for bone and joint health.

Boron, in case you aren't familiar with it, is a common element found in rocks, soil, and water.

Research findings on boron include the following:

- The femur bones and synovial fluid of individuals with osteoarthritis contain much less boron content than people without the disorder.
- Surgeons have observed that the bones of patients using boron supplements are much harder to cut than those of nonsupplemented patients.
- Boron supplementation apparently accelerates the healing of broken bones.
- Boron plays a pivotal regulatory role in the bone metabolism of vitamin D, as well as calcium and magnesium.
- Epidemiological evidence collected by Newnham suggests that in areas of the world where boron intakes are low, there is a higher incidence of arthritis in both animals and humans. Where intakes are higher, the incidence is lower. Newnham believes that excessive use of chemical fertilizers contributes to lower boron content in agricultural soil and, as a consequence, the crops produced in such soil.
- In a double-blind, two-month trial at the Royal Melbourne Hospital involving patients with diagnosed osteoarthritis, seven out of nine

> patients taking daily boron supplements claimed improvement, including significantly less pain, at the conclusion of the two-month trial.

Newnham, who is also an osteopathic physician, is now eighty, and semiretired in England. But he still actively promotes boron as a major preventive and therapeutic strategy for arthritis and osteoporosis. He says that both he and his wife have no symptoms of osteoarthritis.

Boron is not considered an essential mineral for human health as are, for instance, calcium, magnesium, and zinc. Thus, there is no RDA for boron. Forrest H. Nielsen, Ph.D., of the U.S. Department of Agriculture's Grand Forks Human Nutrition Research Center in North Dakota, believes there should be. In a 1998 article in the journal *Biological Trace Mineral Research,* Nielsen argued that the scientific evidence demonstrates "beneficial, if not essential, effects in both animals and humans. Perhaps the best-documented beneficial effect of boron is on calcium metabolism or utilization, thus bone calcification and maintenance."

A significant number of people fail to consistently consume more than 1 milligram of boron daily and this could be of clinical concern, said Nielsen. Boron is found most abundantly in fruits, vegetables, legumes, and nuts.

Curtiss D. Hunt, Ph.D., a research biologist and colleague of Nielsen's, believes that boron may be beneficial in the control of inflammation. He has launched a study to determine the effects of dietary boron in women suffering from rheumatoid arthritis, a much more inflammatory condition than osteoarthritis.

Although I have no clinical experience with boron, I find the research promising and hope additional studies will be conducted to explore the potential.

How Much Boron to Take

- Human and animal data suggest 1 to 13 grams daily as an acceptable safe range of boron intake for adults. Consumption of a diet high in fruits and vegetables can increase boron intake to around 3 milligrams a day.

Newnham believes that 6 milligrams can have a powerful preventive effect for most people. "But for most of us that much is not available in food so we need a supplement," he says.

For therapy, he recommends 9 milligrams daily. Very heavy people need more. "When symptoms improve, a supplement of 3 milligrams a day will generally prevent their return," he says.

sam-e

Until the spring of 1999, virtually nobody in the United States had ever heard of Sam-e. However, as Judith Horstman of *Arthritis Today* reported, when this European supplement hit the market "it zoomed in a matter of months from an unknown import to one of the top-selling supplements in the country."

Sam-e has been used by doctors in Europe for about twenty years as a treatment for osteoarthritis and depression. Numerous studies indicate the substance relieves pain and depression as effectively as many medications but without any apparent side effects or drug interactions.

Sam-e (short for S-adenosylmethionine) is a fundamental and naturally occurring compound contributing to the body's remarkable enzyme system that is continually converting substances into other substances. This activity is called methylation. Sam-e participates in countless processes, including the production of cartilage, neurotransmitters, cell membranes, and the regulation of hormones. The research shows that Sam-e levels decline in the body as we age, are depressed, or have low levels of B complex vitamins.

Doctors familiar with Sam-e say that it takes about two weeks to feel the benefits.

In the *Arthritis Today* report, some doctors suggest starting with 800 milligrams daily, in two divided doses, for osteoarthritis pain. If improvement in pain or mood is seen within two weeks, the dosage can be reduced to 400 milligrams daily. If no improvement is seen in that time, the doctors suggest increasing the dosage and trying again for two more weeks. Taking a B complex supplement may be helpful, as the B vitamins assist in the utilization of Sam-e.

How Much Sam-e to Take

- The amount of Sam-e used in studies ranges from 200 milligrams to 1,600 milligrams daily, with the higher range used for depression.

magnesium

Most people, according to surveys, are deficient in the mineral magnesium, and therein lies a great deal of unrecognized suffering in our society.

According to Mildred Seelig, Ph.D., author of a major medical textbook on the magnesium-disease connection and an adjunct professor of family and preventive medicine at Emory University in Atlanta, all stress and trauma, whether physical or emotional, causes a loss of the body's stores of magnesium. "And if you don't have enough magnesium to begin with, you run the risk of more serious reactions," she says.

Stress includes overwork, too much exercise or physical activity, mental or emotional duress, surgery or trauma, and chronic pain.

The typical magnesium-deficient American diet means there is little magnesium on reserve to deal with stressful situations. The low magnesium compounds the effects of the original stress. "In essence, you are creating a second front of stress and thus you have intensification of stress reactions," says Seelig. "Without adequate magnesium, and the life-supporting activities it contributes to in the body, events can dramatically become life-threatening."

The mineral is a major partner in more than three hundred enzymatic reactions in the body, including the generation of cellular energy and muscle relaxation, the synthesis of fat, protein, and nucleic acids, and the maintenance of strong bones. It enhances calcium absorption in the body. Deficiency is involved in a wide range of symptoms, from muscle cramps and spasms, tics and tremors, premenstrual difficulties, back pain, bone deterioration, and chest pain to life-threatening convulsions, arrhythmias, and heart attacks.

Vegetables, nuts, and whole grains are rich in magnesium, but most Americans don't eat enough of these. The national preference for processed foods ensures a risky low-magnesium intake. The refining of whole grains eliminates most of the magnesium content. For example, the processing of whole wheat to white flour causes a magnesium loss of 82 percent.

High-fat diets also have a negative effect on magnesium. The fat forms soaps in the gut that wash out whatever magnesium is contained in the food. High-fat diets thus markedly increase the requirement for magnesium. Anyone who regularly consumes alcoholic beverages is undoubtedly deficient in magnesium. Even a small amount drains magnesium. Colas and other soft-drinks rich in phosphates inactivate magnesium. Some parts of the country, notably the southeast, have low levels of magnesium in drinking water.

Research on bone density and osteoporosis in women has emphasized calcium and vitamin D. However, we need to think also in terms of other minerals that are important for strong bones, such as magnesium and boron. We take in too much calcium and too little magnesium. Magnesium is needed to balance calcium. When I constantly hear doctors raising concern about women in particular not getting enough calcium to create strong bones, I wish they would also mention magnesium and other minerals that are frequently deficient in our diets. Current recommendations call for a calcium to magnesium ratio that is too high in the opinion of many experts. Many nutritionally oriented physicians think the ratio should be two to one, or even one to one.

I am bringing up the issue of magnesium because I think it so important to overall health, including joint health, even though researchers have not found any direct links to osteoarthritis. I routinely recommend magnesium to my patients.

Magnesium does play a role in relaxing muscles. The muscle cramps and spasms suffered by many individuals are often the result of low magnesium. If muscles constantly remain tight, they may create unhealthy forces on joints that contribute to wear and tear. Magnesium also reduces tissue swelling and may reduce the swelling in the joints.

Epsom salts is a good old-fashioned way of helping aching joints. I suggest to many of my pain patients that they pour Epsom salt crystals into a hot bathtub until they do not dissolve anymore, creating a supersaturated solution. Then soak in the tub. Epsom salt, magnesium sulfate, has been a musculoskeletal remedy for hundreds of years.

How Much Magnesium to Take

- Slowly build up to 300 or 400 milligrams or more a day, in the form of magnesium aspartate or magnesium glycinate.

If you take too much magnesium you may experience a laxative effect. So start slowly with perhaps 50 or 100 milligrams twice a day. If you have never taken magnesium, you may experience some temporary gas in the beginning.

For individuals who are physically very active or exposed to considerable stress, the amount can be increased.

combinations

Today, the supplement marketplace is filled with a variety of joint health formulas. For the most part, these combinations don't have track records of long-term use or research, whereas many of the individual ingredients they contain probably do. Typically, supplement manufacturers put together compounds known to have positive effects on the joints, such as glucosamine, chondroitin, MSM, boswellia, and various herbs. The rationale is that if one ingredient is helpful, two or more may work better by addressing different aspects of joint physiology. Such combinations may indeed provide added value and firepower.

There is nothing wrong with trying a combination if the ingredients look good to you. Just remember, your body is the ultimate laboratory. If a particular product works for you and causes no side effects, well and good.

Following are a number of studies on combination supplements:

- A combination of glucosamine HCL (1,500 milligrams daily), chondroitin sulfate (1,200 milligrams), and a buffered (nonacid) form of vitamin C called manganese ascorbate (228 milligrams) relieved symptoms of knee arthritis in a sixteen-week trial among thirty-four U.S. Navy personnel.
- Another study with the patented formula Cosamin (1,000 milligrams of glucosamine, 800 milligrams of chondroitin, and 152 milligrams of magnesium ascorbate) was also found to be effective for

more than half of seventy-two patients with mild to moderate osteoarthritis of the knee. They showed significant improvement after four and six months. Patients with severe osteoarthritis did not show significant improvement.

- Wesley E. Shankland, DDS, Ph.D., of Columbus, Ohio, a specialist in facial and cranial pain, tested a combination of glucosamine, chondroitin, and vitamin C among fifty new patients with osteoarthritis of the temporomandibular joint (TMJ). Within two weeks, forty patients reported a decrease in TMJ joint "noises" along with a reduction in pain and swelling. About 8 percent reported no noticeable change, and 10 percent did not comply with the study protocol. Shankland's patients used 1,600 milligrams of glucosamine HCL, 1,200 milligrams of chondroitin sulfate, and 1,000 milligrams of calcium ascorbate (another buffered form of vitamin C) twice daily.
- At the 1998 scientific meeting of the American College of Rheumatology, the successful use of a combination of four traditional Ayurvedic herbs from India was reported. The four are ginger, turmeric, boswellia, and ashwagandha. In a double-blind study involving ninety patients with osteoarthritis, 50 percent of the participants experienced significant and sustained pain relief. Each of these plant substances have a long history of use for arthritis in India. Some of them are frequently used in combination with glucosamine and MSM.

THE ARTHRITIS PREVENTION SUPPLEMENT PROGRAM

The following supplements should be used on a *daily basis* as part of an overall program to protect your joints.

If you experience any discomfort from a particular supplement, reduce the dosage or stop taking it.

If you cannot find a supplement in exactly the same dose I recommend, don't be concerned. Purchase the nearest potency.

Reminder: Supplements are not meant to replace good food. Improve your diet first.

Step 1

- A high-quality multivitamin and mineral formula
- Vitamin C—at least 500 milligrams
- Glucosamine—1,500 milligrams
- Chondroitin sulfate—1,200 milligrams
- MSM—up to 3,000 milligrams

You can generally find higher-quality and state-of-the-art products in health-food stores. However, remember the warning on glucosamine and chondroitin products earlier in the chapter.

All multivitamin and mineral formulas contain some vitamin C. If the amount is less than 500 milligrams you may want to add more separately. A multi will often contain adequate vitamin D.

Step 2

- Omega-3 fatty acids—follow label instructions
- Boron—up to 6 milligrams daily
- Vitamin B6—100 milligrams
- Vitamin E—400 IUs
- Magnesium—100 milligrams to start

Take these supplements also on a daily basis but add them to your program at the rate of one per week. This will give your body ample time to adjust to each supplement and will allow you to monitor for any possible reaction.

Your multi will contain some vitamin B6, E, and magnesium, put probably not as much as I recommend here. You can add the additional amounts last, after the fatty acid and boron supplements, which are not likely to be part of a multi formulation.

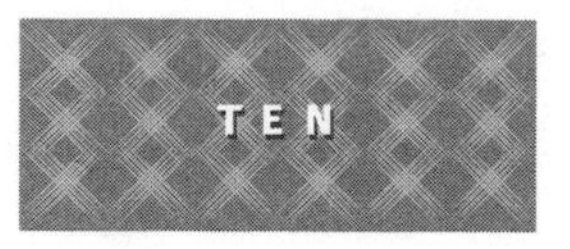

Water Your Thirsty Joints

David Brownstein, M.D., suffered from asthma until six years ago, when he heard a doctor lecture about how many health problems can be caused by not drinking enough water.

Brownstein, who practices in West Bloomfield, Michigan, and is an assistant clinical professor of medicine at Wayne State University, realized that he was drinking hardly any water. Could his body, as the lecturer described, be in a state of dehydration? Could his asthma symptoms be related?

Brownstein was intrigued by the notion of dehydration as a major factor in the cause of asthma. At the time, he was using numerous inhalers to control his symptoms.

"Upon increasing my water intake, I noticed an immediate improvement," he says. "The water helped my asthma and my allergies immediately. I was able to stop using the inhalers within six weeks. Now I rarely use any medication for my asthma. My symptoms are almost totally gone."

This amazing personal experience inspired Brownstein to start recommending "water therapy" to the patients in his holistic medical practice. "The results have been astounding," he says. "I see significant improvement in my patients for many different conditions simply by telling patients to drink more water. I now routinely ask new patients how much water they drink. The typical answer is little or none."

One such patient was a seventy-three-year-old woman with moderate osteoarthritis of the knees. She was taking anti-inflammatories for the pain when Brownstein first saw her in early 1999.

"At the time of her initial visit we did a number of lab tests," he says. "I told her to return in about two months, at which time I would review the tests and design an individual therapeutic program for her. Until then, I told her to increase her water intake. When she returned, she had stopped all her medications. She said that the pain, swelling, and heat in the knee joint resolved in about six weeks. Today she is virtually pain free on a wholistic program that includes keeping up her water intake."

"Her experience is typical," says Brownstein. "Patients report pain relief and more mobility. Almost everybody improves to some extent, some substantially, and I have used it now for hundreds of patients. Frequently they are able to lower the amount of medication they need to take, and in some cases even discontinue the medication."

There is no question in his mind that people with osteoarthritis improve as soon as they increase their water intake if they are not drinking enough water to begin with—and most of them aren't. Moreover, he believes that if you are dehydrated, you will not improve without increasing your water intake.

"I tell my patients that many of the natural remedies I recommend won't work unless they increase their water intake first," he says. "Sometimes we don't have to do anything else but that. Just increase their drinking water.

"When patients first come to see me we take a detailed medical history and perform a variety of blood work and lab tests. I don't set up their treatment program until they come back for a second visit, usually six to eight weeks later. At the time of the first visit I ask them about water intake and strongly recommend they drink an ample amount of water every day. The great majority of them are already significantly improved when they return, just from increasing their water intake. I know the water is effective because I haven't treated them yet."

Brownstein says it generally takes about four weeks to experience improvement. "That's how long it takes to rehydrate the body and for the cells to adjust to the increased water content."

Most of his patients, the Michigan physician learned, were previously drinking sodas, coffee, or tea. "They are definitely not the same as water," he says. "These other beverages have ingredients which do not enable the body to utilize them the same way as it does water, the body's natural, evolutionary beverage. Some of the things we drink are diuretics, that is, they cause the body to excrete more liquid or block the absorption of water. Coffee, for instance, is a diuretic. Sugar also has a diuretic-like effect. And sodas are loaded with sugar."

When Brownstein tells other doctors about his experience with water, they usually just laugh it off. "But I am not laughing, and neither are my patients," he says. "They are very surprised and very pleased."

Brownstein believes that a simple water program is applicable to both prevention and treatment of arthritis. "This is a wonderful, simple technique that resolves a common and unheralded problem of dehydration in our society. Not only does it work for arthritis, but it also helps normalize blood pressure and certainly cures a lot of constipation. There is usually some improvement in all conditions."

How's Your Water Level?

- You are 75 percent water. Your brain is 85 percent water.
- You lose nearly six pints of water a day: a pint in perspiration, two pints in breathing out, and three pints in urine.
- Are you replacing what you lose?

"dr. batman" and research into diseases of dehydration

The lecturer speaking on water who inspired Dr. Brownstein was Fereydoon Batmanghelidj, M.D., of Falls Church, Virginia, the author of an eye-opening book entitled *Your Body's Many Cries for Water* (Falls Church, VA: Global Health Solutions). Batmanghelidj (pronounced Batman-gay-lij," or as many Americans call him, "Dr. Batman"), has studied the effects of water (or lack of it) in the human body for more than twenty years. He believes that many of today's serious illnesses are caused by chronic dehydration of the body.

The London-trained physician's interest in water goes back to his native Iran, where he was jailed as a political prisoner from 1979 to 1982. When fellow prisoners asked him to help another man suffering from an acute peptic ulcer attack, all he had to offer was water. He gave the man two glasses of water. To his surprise, the prisoner's pain vanished in minutes. During the next two years, as one of the prison's doctors, Batmanghelidj researched and applied the use of water for treating people under stress. A clinical report describing his treatment of more than three thousand peptic ulcer cases with water appeared in a 1983 issue of the *Journal of Clinical Gastroenterology.*

Since his prison experience, he has devoted his full-time attention to researching, writing, and lecturing about dehydration-related health problems.

"My understanding from research is that pain is mostly a symptom of dehydration at the site of wherever the pain is felt," he says. "And if you have chronic pain in the spine, hands, or legs, that means those joints are thirsting for water. You are not drinking enough water. The pain is due to dehydrated joints, plus wear and tear, and the inability of the cartilage to repair the damage.

"Nobody ever speaks about lack of water as a contributing factor for osteoarthritis but it is only logical if you understand that the cartilage surfaces of bones in a joint contain much water. The lubricating property of this 'held water' allows the two opposing surfaces to freely glide over one another during joint movement.

"In a well-hydrated cartilage, the rate of friction damage is minimal. In a dehydrated cartilage, the rate of 'abrasive' damage is increased. The ratio between the rate of regeneration of cartilage cells to their 'abrasive peel' is an indicator of their joint efficiency."

How does fluid get to the joints? Batmanghelidj says that in a well-hydrated body, water is carried by the blood into bones and diffuses throughout the bone tissue and marrow. At the bone ends it is absorbed into the base attachment of cartilage for uptake into the cartilage tissue. When the body lacks adequate water, this normal route of water to the cartilage dries up. The serum is too concentrated to diffuse and seep normally through the tiny vessels in the tissues and into the cartilage. In compensation, the body "pumps" extra circulation into the joint capsule. However, this route doesn't bring the necessary fluid into the cartilage tissue where water is needed for the production of new cartilage. Instead it acts as a temporary lubricant for the joint capsule, but in the process creates inflammation, stiffness, and pain.

Batmanghelidj believes that pain is produced by the dilation of the small blood vessels carrying an extraordinary load of fluid to the joint capsule and as well by the actual expansion of the capsule from the introduction of the extra fluid. "Joint surfaces have nerve endings that regulate all functions," and they now produce signals of pain, he says.

Pain is also created by the accumulation of local acidity and toxic substances in the surrounding tissues, he adds. A normal amount of hydration washes out the acidity and toxins.

"The environment of cartilage is alkaline," he explains. "In dehydration, it becomes acid. The acidity sensitizes the nerve endings, and they register this drastic change by producing pain. The cartilage cells, which depend on adequate water, sense the drought, and send out alarm signals of pain, because they would soon die and peel off from their contact surfaces if the dehydrated state continues."

And yet another connection with pain is the effect of dehydration on the status of the serotonin system in the body, he says. Serotonin is a neurotransmitter, a hormonelike substance produced by the nervous system that is involved in our behavior and mood. One of Batmanghelidj's research premises is that dehydration contributes to a low serotonin level, which in turn results in a person becoming depressed and feeling more pain.

In any case, initial pain must be treated with a "regular increase in water intake," he contends. The increase in water will rehydrate the cartilage through the bone tissue—the normal bone route of water and serum diffusion to the cartilage.

If this isn't done, dehydration continues in the cartilage, preventing proper repair, replacement, and "slipperyness" of cartilage. "Prolonged local drought leaves the cartilage short of water, produces a more-than-normal amount of friction and shearing stress, the surfaces of the joints become increasingly rough and ragged in response to the forces applied, and osteoarthritis eventually becomes established," he says.

In Batmanghelidj's view, injury thus occurs to the cartilage not just by wear and tear but by the lack of sufficient water as well. He believes, in fact, that dehydration often precedes the wear and tear, creating an environment in the cartilage tissue that promotes damage.

"If pain occurs in more than one joint and on both sides of the body, it indicates that the brain assesses the strain to be equal for all joints and assumes these joints are not fully prepared to endure a particular level of pressure until one or all of them are fully hydrated," he contends. "This type of pain also needs to be addressed with a regular increase in water intake until cartilage is fully hydrated. To avoid disfigurement, one should take the very initial pain seriously and regard it as an SOS call by the joint for more water. You need to increase your water intake. If the pain does not disappear after some days of adequate water intake and repeated gentle bending of the joints to bring more circulation to the area, one should consult a doctor."

the water–back pain connection

Dr. Batmanghelidj also sees drought in the body as a major contributor to lower back pain. He points out that the disks separating the spinal vertebrae support 75 percent of the weight of your upper body mass. The spinal disks have unique hydraulic properties that absorb and hold water in their central cores. They become, in effect, "water cushions."

"The discs, when fully hydrated, act as wedges and shock absorbers between the vertebrae," he says. "They get continuously squeezed of their water by the pressure of the body mass above each disk that the disk has to support. Through a suction force created by a local vacuum effect, the disks again absorb the water squeezed out of them and expand to fully pack the vertebral joint. In a dehydrated state, when the body mass constantly squeezes out the water content of the disks during movement and bending, not enough of the lost water can be replaced. Dehydrated discs with their shrunken cores gradually become less supportive of the weight of the body. They lose their wedge and shock-absorbing quality and the spinal joints become less firm."

When this occurs, Batmanghelidj adds, "the muscles of the back have to work proportionately harder to hold the body upright. The overworked muscles gradually become fatigued and begin to spasm. It is the spasm of the muscles that creates back pain in 80 percent of cases. The muscles in spasms also have an increased toxic waste content that cannot be washed away because of local dehydration, thus generating additional pain."

The doctor's recommendation for back pain? You guessed it. Drink more water! For sciatica as well, and many other conditions.

"Basically, whatever the illness you may have, try water before anything else," he says. "Drink enough water in the first place and you may not have an illness."

For more information about his books and videos on healing with water, see the resources listed at the end of this chapter.

I agree with Batmanghelidj when he laments the fact that there is no research on the use of water as a simple yet effective form of treatment and medication. "Everyone runs away from water as a field of research," he says. "The problem is that water is free and widely available and doesn't fit into the commercialization, business, and profitability practices of our medical system."

I have long recommended to my patients to drink an adequate amount of fluids, and particularly water, and to make it a conscious part of their daily routines. I tell my patients to drink eight fluid ounces every hour and if they miss an hour to double up the next hour. I have indeed found that pain problems are helped by water and made worse when a patient is dehydrated or hardly drinks water at all.

I recall the case of a cousin of mine who had developed aches and pains and other health problems about twenty years ago. He was a professor of psychology and learned about the use of water for healing purposes. He became a "heavy drinker" (of water) and subsequently reported that his symptoms disappeared.

Water indeed has both preventive and healing properties . . . and also keeps the skin looking young and the bowels functioning better. The traditional doctor's recommendation to drink a lot of fluids is certainly well founded. In fact, if you heed it you may not find yourself in the doctor's office as much. As Thoreau said, "Water is the only drink for a wise man." Just make sure you're getting enough.

Dr. Batman's Water Formula

Dr. Batman offers the following formula for both preventive and therapeutic water intake:

- Drink half your body weight in ounces of water, as pure as possible, throughout each day. Thus, if you weigh 150 pounds, drink seventy-five ounces. That is the equivalent of about ten eight-ounce glasses.

- Add a quarter-teaspoon of sea salt for each quart of water. There are thirty-two fluid ounces (four glasses) per quart. Why add salt? Sodium is a major component of bone tissue and vital for joint health. Cartilage retains a considerable amount of sodium to remain properly hydrated, and sodium helps maintain the proper alkalinity of cartilage tissue.
- Coffee, tea, and alcohol are not forms of water. As a matter of fact, they are drying agents, and push water out of the body.
- During the summer and periods of humidity, or when involved in a vigorous exercise program, you need more water than normal, up to fifteen or even more glasses a day.
- Drink a half-hour before eating to prepare the stomach for its digestive functions.

Resources

The books *Your Body's Many Cries for Water, How to Deal with Back Pain & Rheumatoid Joint Pain,* and *ABC of Asthma, Allergies and Lupus,* by Fereydoon Batmanghelidj, M.D., are available through Global Health Solutions, P.O. Box 3189, Falls Church, VA 22043 (phone: 703-848-2333). Videotapes on water therapy are also available. For more information on Dr. Batmanghelidj's work, visit his website at *www.watercure.com.*

For more details on Dr. Brownstein's experience using water and other methods for arthritis, you can obtain his book *Overcoming Arthritis* by calling Medical Alternatives Press at 888-647-5616 or by visiting his website at *www.drbrownstein.com*. Brownstein has also written about water therapies and other holistic treatments in his book *The Miracle of Natural Hormones,* likewise available from Medical Alternatives Press.

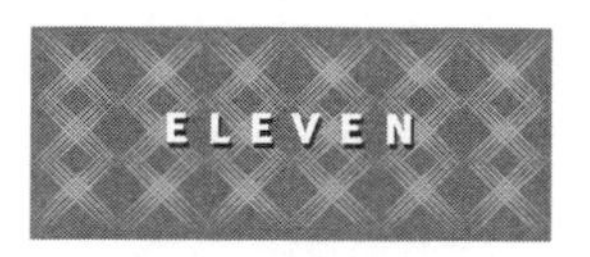

Keep Your Joints Flexible with Yoga

The ancient Indian practice of yoga is valued throughout the world not only for its ability to develop spirituality, but also for its ability to promote physical, mental, and emotional health, and to relieve pain and stress. According to very old texts that have survived the passage of time, arthritis is among the conditions that are benefited.

I have long recommended yoga to my patients as a prevention strategy as well as an avenue for obtaining relief from arthritis.

In recent years, the health-boosting and stress-busting benefits of yoga have been recognized by the medical mainstream. In the late 1990s a number of U.S. medical insurance companies, such as Blue Cross and Mutual of Omaha, introduced yoga into their wellness programs. And for good reason. Yoga is the perfect way to stretch your body, an ancient method that has survived the test of time because it works so well. The systemic stretching routines of yoga represent a powerful anti arthritis tool.

Yoga promotes a healing mode in the body by maintaining good muscle tone and joint flexibility. Moreover, it opens clogged channels throughout the body and improves the circulation, thus bringing vital nutrients and oxygen to all the tissues, including the joints. The mechanical actions of stretching and compressing of body tissues created by the practice of yoga may even affect the permeability of cells in a positive way and help stimulate metabolic processes inside.

In an article published in the February 2000 issue of *Rheumatic*

Disease Clinics of North America, researchers at Philadelphia's Hahnemann University and the University of Pennsylvania School of Medicine suggest that correctly supervised yoga may provide the motion and forces on joints needed to preserve integrity. Marian Garfinkel, Ed.D., and H. Ralph Schumacher, Jr., M.D., pointed out in their journal paper that there is a growing understanding of how mechanical actions can alter cell function and protect cartilage tissue that is lost by immobilization. "Effects of mechanical and fluid pressure on structures such as cartilage . . . suggest that yoga postures might alter joint function," they wrote.

Over the years I have often referred patients to Larry Payne, Ph.D., an internationally renowned yoga instructor. Larry is chairman of the International Association of Yoga Therapists, a coauthor of *Yoga for Dummies,* and a cofounder of the yoga program at the UCLA Medical School, where medical students are learning the ancient practice. The program is the first of its kind at a major university medical center in the United States and was inspired by Richard Usatine, M.D., the school's assistant dean of student affairs. Usatine went to Payne for help after standard medical treatment failed to help back pain resulting from an automobile accident. The yoga techniques that he learned provided such significant relief that Payne was invited to teach UCLA medical students.

"I hope that this exposure will carry through their careers and allow them to have a much more open mind in other ways of treating patients," Usatine told a reporter.

I asked Payne to share an easy-to-do program of arthritis prevention for beginners, similar to the beginning movements he teaches to corporate executives, athletes, and celebrities, and in his group sessions. You will be amazed at how effective these simple movements are. And you can actually do many of them lying down or sitting comfortably in a chair!

If you are interested in going beyond these few simple movements, refer to Larry's book or his "*User-Friendly Yoga*" videos, or other widely available books and videos, or seek out a qualified yoga instructor in your area.

LARRY PAYNE'S USER-FRIENDLY YOGA PROGRAM FOR ARTHRITIS PREVENTION

The goal of yoga is not to stand on your head but to quiet the distractions of the mind and allow your awareness to enter higher states of consciousness. You want to sit quietly to do that, and in order to facilitate the process, yoga offers many different postures to eliminate stress, improve strength, flexibility, and circulation, and create a healing mode in the mind and body. Different postures affect different parts, systems, and conditions.

The breath is very important in this process. We want to slow down the breath by breathing through the nose. Unless you have an obstruction, this is the way to breathe. Through your nose. Both the inhale and the exhale. This also warms and filters the air.

There are four parts to the yoga breath. A comfortable inhale. Pause. A long comfortable exhale. Then pause.

Gradually take longer and smoother breaths. Focus on your breath. Don't practice these exercises while watching television or listening to the radio. The word *yoga* in Sanskrit means "union," and in this situation we are talking about union between body, breath, and mind. You can't create a union while you watch TV. You must be in the moment and not distracted.

As you slow down the breath, you slow down the heartbeat. That's like sending a fax to your nervous system to calm down and relax.

Let the breath be your de-stressor. Keep in mind that 80 percent of our illnesses are stress related. So whether you are interested in prevention or healing, you should attend to stress reduction first.

For exercises involving movements of the limbs, keep the limbs "soft." Don't lock them or keep them rigid. Be relaxed. "Soft" limbs enable the spine to move more readily.

The first five steps can be done in five to ten minutes. It may not seem that you are doing much, but you are. In these few exercises you are activating the healing effect of the breath as well as moving the largest appendages (the arms and legs), their joints, and connected muscles. All these movements exercise the spine as well in a gentle, yet fundamental way. The spine should always be warmed up in this way, with flexion and extension.

If you have the time and desire, I have added more steps that can enhance both a preventive and healing program.

Wear comfortable clothing when doing these movements. The ancient tradition calls for practicing yoga at sunrise and sunset. That doesn't always work in our modern age. So do it at a convenient time, once or twice a day, as long as it is not after eating.

Step 1. Breathing for Stress Reduction

Lie down on your back (preferably), or sit comfortably on the floor or in a chair. Focus your attention on your breath as you comfortably inhale and exhale through your nose.

You will notice that the breath moves your body. For instance, it moves the joints in your spine. And much of the arthritis we have involves the spine. When you inhale, your body arches and the spine opens. When you exhale, your spine contracts along with all the connected muscles and ligaments.

The rest of what you do in yoga follows the breath. It acts as the current in the river, moving you along as you swim. Anything that has to do with healing or good yoga practice should include a conscious focus on the breathing movement itself.

The key to using breath as a pain reliever is long exhales. The exhale phase of the breath is the calming and quieting part.

In this opening position, as you lie on your back, bend your knees at a 90-degree angle, and rest your heels on a chair or foot rest. Cover your eyes with a towel. Your arms are extended down along your sides, or your hands are folded comfortably on your belly.

As you settle down and relax and dissolve tension, you are priming yourself to get the benefits from all the other movements that follow.

Time of exercise: two and a half minutes to five minutes.

Step 2. Lying Arm Raise

You're still on your back. Now add movement, beginning with your arms. As you inhale, raise your arms and hands forward and up over your head. Then bring them down to the floor in an extended position beyond your head. The backs of your hands are comfortably resting on the floor.

Pause. And as you exhale, follow with the return movement by bringing the arms back to the starting position.

One of the most common sites of tension are neck and shoulders, the area between the shoulder blades. Just by "waving" your arms in this simple back and forth movement, you are releasing that tension. You are also "warming up" and stretching the spine.

This exercise can also be done sitting in a chair. You raise your arms forward, up, and overhead.

Repetitions: six to ten times.

Step 3. Lying Bent-Leg Extension

You're on your back—still. The knees are bent and the feet flat on the floor. As you exhale, bring your knees up toward your chest. Hold the back of the thighs with your hands, each hand on one thigh.

Once in this starting position, start the movement. Inhale and raise your feet up overhead. Keep holding the backs of the thighs with your hands.

Pause. Start your exhalation. Bring your feet back down by bending the knees and bringing your heels down comfortably toward the buttocks.

Repetitions: six to ten times.

Step 4. The Bridge

You are still on your back. Your arms are at your sides, palms downward. The knees are bent, the feet flat on the floor at hip width.

Inhale and raise your hips as high as you can comfortably bring them. Pause.

Exhale and lower the hips back down to the floor.

Repetitions: six to ten times.

Step 5. Belly Breathing

Repeat the breathing, as in step one, or relax in some other way.

Step 6, The Rejuvenation Sequence

You are in a standing position, with feet apart (at hip width) and arms at your sides.

Inhale and slowly raise your arms out from the sides and upward over your head.

Pause.

Then, as you exhale, bend forward from the waist. Bring your head downward and toward your knees. Your hands come forward and downward toward the floor. Start the movement with your legs straight. When you feel a pull, and the muscles tightening in the back of the legs, soften and slightly bend the knees. Remember to keep your arms and legs soft, not rigid.

Pause. Bend your knees more, if necessary, to be comfortable.

With your next inhale, sweep your arms upward and outward as if you had wings. Your arms are now extended outward at about shoulder height. Your palms are facing down. Lift your head up a bit. Try to create a saddlelike curve in your lower back.

Pause.

Now exhale. Float your arms, hands, head, and torso down again in the direction of the floor.

Now as you inhale, slowly bring your torso all the way up again to an erect position. At the same time, sweep your arms up, out, and extended over your head.

Pause.

Finally, exhale and lower your arms back to the sides in the starting position.

Repetitions: six to eight times.

The function of this classical pose is to stretch, strengthen, and improve the flexibility of your spine and the backs of your legs. It also benefits the joints of the hands, arms, and legs.

Step 7. Twist

Lie on your back. Arms are extended outward to the sides at shoulder level, forming a T. The knees are bent with the feet flat on the floor. The heels are as comfortably close to your buttocks as possible.

Take a deep breath. Exhale and allow your knees to rotate laterally to the right and as far down toward the floor as possible. At the same time, rotate your head to the left. Pause.

Inhale and return to the starting position. Pause.

Exhale, and now move your knees to the left and down, and rotate your head to the right.

This exercise helps to rejuvenate the spine—from top to bottom—and improve flexibility.

Repetitions: six to ten times.

After you complete the repetitions for this twisting movement, continue to lie on your back. Then, as you exhale, bring your knees upward and hold the backs of your thighs, as in step 3. Hold in this comfortable position for six to eight breaths.

yoga for computer users

Long hours of work at the computer can create considerable tension and muscle fatigue in the upper back and neck. To prevent or relieve the tension, and to head off chronic problems, Larry Payne offers two simple routines. Do them several times a day, or whenever you take a brief break. You can alternate the exercises, but if you have to choose between the two, the second is the most effective. If you can do them both, do them in the following order:

Standing Alternating Arm Raise with Head Turn

Stand with your arms hanging at your sides.

As you inhale, bring your right arm up and overhead, and turn your head to the left.

On the exhale, bring the arm back down and turn your head back so you are looking forward.

On the next inhale, bring your left arm up and overhead, and turn your head to the right.

When you exhale, again bring the arm back down and turn the head to a forward position.

Perform four or five repetitions on each side.

This exercise stretches the neck and helps relieve tension in the neck and the muscles of the upper back that extend up into the head.

"Wing and a Prayer"

While standing, press your palms together at chest level, as if you are praying. In yoga, we call this *namaste*. The fingers are pointing upward.

As you inhale, raise the joined hands up and overhead. Raise your chin, bend your neck, and look up at the hands.

Now exhale. As you do, bring the hands back down to the starting position at your chest.

The second part of this exercise also starts from the prayer position. As you inhale, expand your chest outward and upward, arching slightly in the back. Move your hands apart and out to the side as far as they will go. Your elbows are still bent, as in the prayer position, and your hands are now facing forward in the direction you are looking. In this motion you should feel your shoulder blades moving closer together.

As you exhale, bring the hands back together in prayer position. Your chest and shoulder blades relax.

Perform six to eight repetitions.

In this combination routine you are lengthening your spine as you raise your hands and then opening your chest when your hands go wide.

Resources

For a general introduction, read *Yoga for Dummies* (Foster City, CA: IDG Books, 1999), by Georg Feuerstein, Ph.D., and Larry Payne, Ph.D.

Larry Payne has produced two excellent videos: *User-Friendly Yoga for Beginners,* a 28-minute video of easy-to-follow yoga routines to shape up the body and reduce stress, and *User-Friendly Back Yoga,* a 23-minute video of routines for the prevention of lower back problems. Both are available through Samata International, Los Angeles (phone: 800-359-0171; on the Internet at *www.samata.com*).

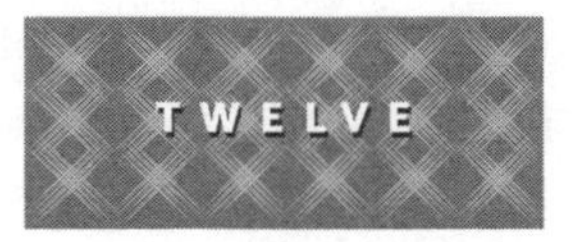

Protect Your Hands

Osteoarthritis affects the hand joints more than any other part of the body. In San Francisco, hand surgeon Robert E. Markison, M.D., sees a good deal of osteoarthritis among patients ranging from aging rock-and-roll drummers to computer workers.

The first joint in the hands to give way to osteoarthritis is often the carpometacarpal joint—also known as the basal joint, located at the base of the thumb, just above the wrist. This pivotal joint is responsible for placing the thumb in countless positions and allowing great freedom of motion in the hand. The function of the thumb and, as a consequence, the hand, has a strong reliance on the integrity of this joint.

Osteoarthritis in this particular joint seems to preferentially affect women, according to researchers. Women have ten to twenty times more arthritis in this site than men. Indeed, says Markison, some 80 percent of his patients are women, and both men and women also frequently develop osteoarthritis in the small joints of the fingers.

"The basal joint is a major trouble spot because it is not a particularly stable joint," says Markison, an associate clinical professor of surgery at the University of California at San Francisco. "The joint receives a tenfold increase of any force transmitted from the thumb tip because of the pulling influences of thumb muscles and tendons. The effect is something like holding up the center pole of a circus tent."

The joint comes relentlessly under siege during a typical day of activity—all pinching and holding actions and everything from lifting a single piece of paper to tapping your thumb against the computer space bar, clutching the mouse, opening a door or a jar of peanut butter, or turning the key in a door. Nearly every aspect of daily living becomes difficult or impossible without a healthy basal joint.

"We develop osteoarthritis of the hands from a combination of heredity and a lifetime of use with longer lifespans," says Markison. "In our contemporary high-speed lifestyle with a broadened scope of the use of the hand in and out of work we are accelerating the aging of the parts, including joints."

It is not possible to connect osteoarthritis of the hands solely to repetitive manual tasks at work, he adds. That's because we don't just use our hands at work, we use them in all our daily activities.

"There is no question that someone with the natural progression of basal arthritis who works all day on the keyboard or who is a musician and practices for many hours, is likely accelerating the disease," explains Markison. "The work activity adds more wear and tear than what would be ordinarily experienced. But does that same person surf the net and clutch a mouse at home? Does that same person ride a mountain bike or play racket sports? That makes it hard to say that the thumb on the space bar or the cello bow was the primary cause.

"We use our hands repetitively and forcefully in and out of work in innumerable ways that create microtraumas to the joints, and all this can contribute to the development of osteoarthritis."

cool hand clue

During more than twenty years in practice, Markison became keenly aware of blood-flow patterns to the hand and specifically that cool hands are a remarkable yardstick in the prevention and treatment of hand problems.

Blood flow per unit of tissue is the determining factor in the maintenance of tissue healing, he explains. Cool hands mean that you don't have a lot of blood flow. As a result, you have less oxygen and nutrients to sustain repetitive or forceful use of the hands. Healing and maintenance depend a great deal on the quality of blood flow.

"It is not a coincidence that most of my upper-limb strain patients have cool hands," Markison says.

Normally, we associate impaired blood flow with cardiovascular problems. Not enough blood to the brain can trigger a stroke. Not enough flow to the heart muscle causes heart attacks.

"And so, too, not enough blood flow to the hands can contribute to repetitive strain problems," Markison points out. "My message is to take remedial action or not take up single tasking, forceful, or repetitive manual work."

How can you tell if you have cool hands?

Just put your hands up to your cheeks.

There may be a connection to osteoarthritis. The nerves, tendons, muscles, and joints of the hands don't feel good in cool-handed people.

hand-saving tips

1. Keep the hands warm, says Markison. This can be accomplished in several ways:
    - The use of fingerless gloves running from the forearms to the middle joints of the fingers. Markison's office recommends Linda Lorraine, a San Francisco glove designer, who offers an array of therapeutic gloves. Her prices start at $15 a pair. For more information, contact Lorraine at 2215 R Market Street #250, San Francisco, CA 94114-1653; phone 415-564-5156; or website *www.feri.com/llgloves.* Lorraine requires a pencil tracing or photocopy of the hand and forearm in order to provide a good fit.
    - Learn biofeedback, visualization, or self-hypnosis techniques that direct attention in a way that can warm the hands.
    - Move to a warmer climate. "People with osteoarthritis feel better if they keep their hands warm," he says.

2. Stay well-hydrated. As we have seen in a previous chapter, adequate water intake is important for both joint and overall health. Markison is a big believer in drinking ample water and routinely recommends two to four quarts daily to patients unless they have a medical contraindication, such as congestive heart failure.

   "My patients, including those with osteoarthritis, do much better on a high water intake," he says. "Being well hydrated translates to better-'oiled' joints. You push microcirculation to the joints and improve the synovial fluid production. I believe that a lack of adequate water aggravates osteoarthritis. Increased water intake also promotes circulation to the fingertips."

3. Be connected from your brain to your fingertips. Be very aware of fixed, odd, twisted postures in your activities. In computer work, for instance, strain is created with the head and limbs forward, and the forearms, wrists, and hands twisted into a palm down position.

   "This defies our evolutionary upright position that emphasizes bringing objects to us, rather than bowing down to them," notes Markison.

4. Perform a simple lymphatic massage. You need good outflow of waste products through the lymphatic system in your hands as well as good inflow of blood through the arteries.

   To help push out waste products, massage from the tips of the fingers up to the elbow with a gentle squeezing action.

   "If the outflow is poor, your hands become a stagnant waste dump," says Markison.

   Do this massage several times a day if possible or whenever you take a break.

5. A good pair of work gloves, with some protective thickness, acts as a buffer against the intense forces exerted on your hand joints whenever you use tools. Gloves can be particularly beneficial for electricians, carpenters, and plumbers, or other individuals whose activities call for repetitive twisting and gripping.

6. Life is based on a balance of rest and activity. Make sure your hands, and all of you, obtain proper rest.

"computeritis"

How you sit and work at the computer can play a role in avoiding or developing repetitive motion injuries such as carpal-tunnel syndrome and muscular strain.

In his hand practice, Robert Markison analyzes the way in which people use their hands in their daily activities, including computer work, and uncovers many problems.

"A lot of people just do things intensely and erroneously and find themselves in deep trouble at a young age, but in addition to that, the major computer makers are failing us," he says. "As chip speeds increase exponentially, we continue to use Human Software and Hardware, Version 1.0. No one guaranteed that the human-information superhighway that runs from the brain to the fingertips and back could tolerate the combining of so many different activities at a single human computer interface.

"We were designed to vary our tasks throughout the day, move around, breathe fresh air, etc. But there are some other important elements of human design that should not be violated. If, as required for computer use, we are in a head-forward position intently staring into the monitor, just three inches of this posture can triple the forces that run through our neck, muscles, and spine.

"If we assume a limb-forward position (like lizards), we tighten up the chest wall (pectoral) muscles that overlie an important part of the human-information superhighway called the brachial plexus.

"This creates downstream consequences that may result in tingling in the hands. If we decide to keep our hands flat on a horizontal plane such as the mouse and keyboard demand (again, lizardlike), we are twisting muscle-tendon units that do not enjoy being twisted.

"Every muscle fiber in the body has an ideal range of length at which it works best. Transgressing these ideal biomechanical patterns leads to some rather unhappy and chronic situations."

Is computering an outright risk factor for osteoarthritis? We don't know yet for sure. The personal computer has been around for less than twenty years and many people have been using it intensely for less than ten. So there are as yet no longitudinal studies to give us answers. In my own clinical experience, long hours at the computer over many years may contribute to osteoarthritis in the neck. Based on his experience, Markison suggests that too much computing runs the risk of accelerating the aging of all tissues, including the joints.

added tips for computer users

In addition to the tips presented above, the following are some computer-specific recommendations that can cut down your risk of developing chronic pain or joint problems if you work at a computer or spend long hours hacking:

- Arrange your equipment so that you can work in a natural and relaxed posture. Adjust everything to find your most effective body postures.
- Adjustable keyboards with split and tilt features help you avoid strained, unnatural positions of the hands. There are also mice available that operate in a more vertical position that again eases hand and upper extremity strain.
- An adjustable chair is essential. Adjustable chairs tend to be more expensive than simple one-position chairs, but the added expense is well worth it. Remember, we all have different sizes and shapes.
- Keep your body in a relaxed yet upright position. The backrest of your chair should support the inward curve of your lower back.
- Arm supports should support the forearms comfortably while typing and at a height that enables shoulders to be relaxed.

- Your keyboard should be located at the height of your elbow, so that your forearm is generally parallel to the floor and at about a 90-degree angle to your upper arm. Your shoulders should not be elevated during keyboard use.

- The hand should be in line with the forearm, a "neutral position." The slope of the keyboard may need to be adjusted so that your wrists are straight, and not bent back, while you type. Type with your hands and wrists "floating" above the keyboard. Use a wrist pad only to rest your wrists between typing. Avoid resting your wrist on sharp edges. Press keys gently—don't bang on them.

- Correct placement of the monitor can reduce eye, shoulder, neck, and upper back strain. Adjust the monitor so that the top of the screen is at or slightly below eye level and right in front of you. The monitor shouldn't be off to the side so that your body or neck is rotated and causing tension. Your eyes should look straight ahead and slightly downward when viewing the middle of the screen.

- Let the shoulder girdle hang loose. Don't work in a shrugged position.

- Proper glasses with the right strength for your work are critical. You don't want to be leaning forward to see the screen clearly. This increases spinal forces and reduces blood flow in the neck and thorax.

- Take as many short breaks as possible. That doesn't mean just stop typing. I mean get your blood pumping. Stretch and move around. (For two very simple yet beneficial yoga postures you can do right at your desk, see chapter 11.)

- Change your posture during the day. Shift your load over different muscles. Even slight changes can make a difference.

- Don't hold your neck in one position for long, even if that is the most comfortable position for you. Try to move your neck frequently as you work at the computer. The body was made to be moved. Every half hour or so, gently turn the chin from one shoulder to the other or move the chin down toward the chest and then upward.

- Consider purchasing voice-recognition software that translates dictation into a microphone connected to the computer directly into a text format. Such software has advanced significantly in recent years to accuracy levels approaching and exceeding 90 percent. Use of voice-recognition software means less use of the hands.

- Improve your physical fitness. Deborah Quilter, the expert on repetitive strain injury whom I referred to in Chapter 5, personally overcame a debilitating condition in her hands. She emphasizes the importance of maintaining physical fitness for jobs that require repetitive motions, including computer work. She, in fact, has created and taught a "computer fitness" program at the New York Health & Racquet Club in Manhattan.

  "So many computer users are sedentary and out of condition," she says. "When you take out-of-condition muscles and use them thousands of times a day, doing the same minute hand movements over and over, you are setting yourself up for a serious injury that starts with a whisper and ends with a scream. Strong muscles help prevent problems. You literally need to become a 'computer athlete' and develop upper-body and back strength. Women in particular need to focus here."

  Also, she adds, "try to limit daily computer use. Too much time at the computer can injure you, even with all the precautions you take."

Resources

Repetitive Strain Injury: A Computer User's Guide (John W. Wiley & Sons, 1994), by Emil Pascarelli, M.D., and Deborah Quilter

The Repetitive Strain Injury Recovery Book (Walker & Company, 1998), by Deborah Quilter.

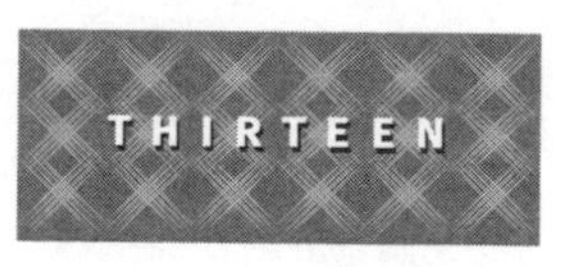

Foot Care—Prevention from the Ground Up

Among other things, Nevada's gambling establishments are famous for the shapely corps of drink servers plying the casino floors. "The image of the sexy cocktail waitress is as vital here as a one-armed bandit," wrote Tom Gorman of the *Los Angeles Times* in a September 2000 article.

However, there's "something of a rebellion afoot," he reported. Cocktail waitresses have united to campaign against the high-heel shoes they must wear on the job.

High-heel-enhanced legs may be pleasing to the male eye, but they are not very pleasing for the females who have to walk on them throughout a long workday. The complaining waitresses, required sometimes to wear heels more than two and a half inches high, are suffering. Many of them regularly take pain medication because of bunions, ingrown toenails, and hammer toes. Some have undergone foot, hip, and back surgeries to correct the "ravages of a career in high heels," the *Times* said.

Indeed, according to the American Podiatric Medical Association, women have four times as many foot problems as men and lifelong patterns of wearing high heels are often the culprit.

High heels also invite lower back pain by increasing the natural (lordotic) curve of the lower spine, thus stressing the muscles in that area. Neurologists and orthopedists treat many women for lower back pain caused by years of everyday high-heel use.

I have long felt that female patients who routinely wear high heels develop osteoarthritis in the knees and back at an earlier age. It was thus with interest that I read a 1998 report in the medical journal *Lancet* that explored the connection between these types of shoes and the joints in the legs. Because osteoarthritis in the knees is twice as common among women as men, the researchers from Harvard's Department of Physical Medicine and Rehabilitation set out to investigate whether damaging torques (forces applied on leg joints) could be caused by high heels.

In the study, twenty fit women were instructed to walk along a platform in bare feet and in heels two and a half inches high. Under the platform, monitoring devices measured the strains and forces on the knee joint as the women went through their paces.

The results showed that the heels created a much higher strain on the knees, and particularly on the inner side of the joint. The researchers noted that osteoarthritis degeneration is known to be more common on the inner side.

"The possibility that wearing high-heeled shoes contributes to osteoarthritis of the knee has not been suggested to date," they said, adding that their study indicates that "the altered forces at the knee caused by walking in high heels may predispose to degenerative changes in the joint."

My hope is that such studies will help bring overdue attention to foot care. It is a sorely neglected area in the consideration of arthritis prevention and treatment. It shouldn't be. Think about it. The feet are the foundation for the rest of the body, and any imbalance can throw the rest of the body out of alignment. This may lead to abnormal wear and tear, aches and pains, fatigue, and degenerative arthritis. Problems in the feet may be felt, as we have seen, in the knees, but also higher up in the hips, back, and even the neck. From a biomechanical standpoint, imbalances that lead to osteoarthritis often start from the ground up—with your feet. And thus your feet are a good place to start when considering prevention. In my practice, I often check the feet first when examining a patient complaining of joint pain.

Osteoarthritis is also very common in any of the twenty-six bones of the foot and ankle and their associated joints. "Frequently, the first place that arthritis develops in the body is the ankle or great-toe joint," says Steve Subotnick, D.P.M., N.D, D.C, of Berkeley, a highly knowledgeable podiatrist, naturopath, and chiropractor with more than thirty years experience treating sports, trauma, and degenerative conditions of the feet.

"Remember that the feet bear the weight of the whole body. Arthritis in the feet is associated with *hallux limitus* (degeneration of the big toe joint), bunions, and heel spurs. Many common problems of the feet often develop into arthritis."

shoe abcs

Many Americans are literally walking on "shaky ground." I am not speaking of earthquakes, but of inappropriate footware. The purpose of shoes is to hold the foot stable as it strikes the ground. But many types of footware, and not only high heels, fail to meet this fundamental criterion.

When I have brought this issue up to patients over the years, some have remarked that Indians only wore moccasins and many people around the world still go barefoot. This is true. However, Indians did not walk on pavement or hard floors. The moccasin protected them from thorns and stones. Actually people who walk barefoot from an early age develop a structurally stronger foot and calluses that appear to provide better protection. The rate of foot problems is lower in populations where shoes are not worn.

I am not pushing a barefoot agenda, but I do believe we have to give more attention to what we put on our feet. Unfortunately, seeing to proper footware for work, leisure, and exercise is a hugely neglected consideration in our society, says Subotnick, a former member of the White House Council on Physical Fitness and Sports, and author of *Sports Medicine of the Lower Extremities* (New York: Churchill Livingstone, 1999).

So, what is proper and what is improper? I asked Subotnick. Here is how he answered:

High Heels

Biomechanically unsound shoes. Your heel is way up high and overloads the ball of your foot. This creates *hallux limitus,* jams the big-toe joints, creates bunions and hammer toes, and wears out the protective fat pad on the bottom of the ball of the feet. In short, they predispose the toes to arthritis.

When you take a foot with a rectangular shape and you shove it into a triangular shoe, that crowds everything together, creating abnormal forces, and after a while, you get arthritis in the joints.

The best advice is to wear high heels only when you have to, such as times when you have to dress up and look good. But carry some sensible shoes with you so that when the feet start hurting you can change. High heels are not meant for walking or for long periods of time. Wearing them regularly for a long time is guaranteed to lead to deformities.

Cowboy boots with narrow, pointed toes and high heels can cause the same kind of problems. But some people claim they are the only shoes that they can wear.

Dress Shoes

Loafers are also a problem. Men persist in wearing Italian-type loafers that have thin leather soles and no shock-absorbing properties. I see many 250-pounders with painful feet who are wearing these beautiful shoes. I tell them to stop. When you walk with these shoes, they simply don't absorb the shock. The thin leather soles are bad for the feet and predispose you to osteoarthritis.

Nowadays, you can purchase dress shoes with a stylish upper look and thicker running-type or rubber soles. Florsheim and Rockport are two American brands that make excellent shoes of this nature. Such shoes absorb 50 percent more shock than a loafer, which doesn't absorb anything. So you are getting much more protection.

Try to wear shoes with thick rubber soles for more support and also with laces that allow you to make the shoes tighter or looser on your feet. Feet may swell some at the end of the day. You can retie the shoes for a looser fit when that happens. You can't do that with a loafer.

RUNNING SHOES

These are usually the best for your feet, and offer the most support. The manufacturers have done their research. Their products are pretty much on a par with each other. Always make sure that there is a finger's width between the end of your longest toe and the front of the shoe.

SANDALS

Sandals with arches, such as Birkenstock and Teva, are excellent. They have good shock absorbing arches. Even the cheap ones "made in China" are OK, as long as they have an arch.

HIKING BOOTS

These are very well constructed. The lightweight hiking books are superb for people with weak ankles, offering a good deal of support.

Small Shoes = Big Trouble

Carol Frey, M.D., of the UCLA Orthopaedic Foot and Ankle Center, conducted a study of 356 healthy women and found that 80 percent of them complained of significant foot pain while wearing shoes. Examination revealed that three-quarters of the women had one or more forefoot deformities.

Further investigation revealed that 88 percent of the women were wearing shoes that were narrower than their feet, by an average of 1.2 centimeters, or about ½ inch. Although individuals with no pain also were found to be wearing too narrow shoes, the average discrepancy in their case was only 0.56 centimeters, or about ¼ inch.

"It is clear," Frey wrote in a medical journal, "that the majority of women wear shoes that are too small for their feet and suffer resultant pain and deformities." Women have 9-to-1 odds of developing various forefoot problems. "Males wear more 'healthy' shoes [that provide] a roomier, nonconstricting environment for the foot than fashion shoes for females."

non-shoe causes of arthritis

Improper footware is one major contributor to osteoarthritis in the feet and elsewhere, but obviously not the only cause. Steve Subotnick cites the following additional foot-related factors:

Congenital Misalignments

The joints are aligned improperly so that instead of taking symmetrical loads they take asymmetrical or eccentric loads, creating irregular joint wear and tear. You may have a leg discrepancy, for instance, where one leg is longer than the other, or one foot flatter than the other. There are a whole variety of misalignments that can be best determined through a consultation with a podiatrist.

If you have a low arch and your heel sags to the outside, you are basically putting weight on half of the joint instead of distributing it evenly throughout the joint. So you wear out the half where most of the weight is being carried. If you have a flat foot (very low arch) you will tend to put more weight on the inside of the joint. If you have a high arch, you may tend to put more weight on the outside of the ankle joint.

Parents can help their children develop a good arch by allowing them to go barefoot as much as is safe and possible.

Good sandals and tennis shoes (see Shoe ABCs above) are the best types of footware. Children do well with good, loose-fitting tennis shoes. Be sure to change shoes often. Kids wear them out fast.

If a child's foot seems abnormal in some way, take the child for an evaluation by a podiatrist. You may be able to prevent some future suffering. Children may need an extra support to help the feet develop normally while the bones are still soft.

A very low arch will benefit from such correction. You can tell the arch is abnormally low when, for instance, a youngster comes out of a swimming pool, walks on the cement, and you can see the water print of the whole foot. In a normal foot, you would see no water print in the area of the arch. This poor foot structure could lead to abnormal joint wear and osteoarthritis down the line.

Pronation, where the big toes bend abnormally inward instead of pointing straight ahead, is another problem that could set the stage for arthritis in later life. This situation causes abnormal stresses on the knee joints. Over decades, this can lead to arthritis of the knees.

If you don't develop your arches, and your feet pronate too much, the risk increases for arthritis in the feet, ankles, and knees. Problems with knees often have to be corrected by using orthotics in the shoes. This often stops the progression of arthritis in the knees.

Obesity

Osteoarthritis in the feet is a particular problem for overweight individuals, says the American Podiatric Medical Association. The reason is that there are so many joints in the feet, and the additional weight contributes to deterioration of cartilage and the development of bone spurs. The combination of misalignments and obesity increases the risk of arthritis.

Chronic Repetitive Stress

Hallux limitus, osteoarthritis of the first metatarsal—phalangeal joint (the big toe knuckle), is a common problem among welders, plumbers, electricians, and carpet layers who constantly squat in their work. Ballet dancers develop it from going on point. Any kind of athletes who do a lot of jumping, such as gymnasts, or long-distance runners who put their feet through years of pounding, also have a high risk for this condition.

Ballet and sports have their inherent risks. Prevention measures include balanced workouts and, in the case of sports, using the best quality shoes with custom-made orthotics appropriate for the body type and activity. There are many different types and styles of orthotics. One orthotic will not serve all functions for active people involved in multiple sports, for instance.

Cross-training can serve to develop good dynamic muscle stability to protect the joints. Strong muscles absorb shock and protect the joints. Fatigued muscles offer little protection and the shock goes to the bone and joints—and leads to osteoarthritis.

Stay on softer surfaces whenever possible.

And retire soon enough to stay out of trouble.

Trauma

Arthritis typically develops after accidents involving fractures of the joints. Surgery or infection can also lead to arthritis. I see this in all the major joints of the feet. The degeneration can develop soon after trauma, or many years afterward.

After trauma, once the fracture has been anatomically reduced, start range-of-motion exercises as soon as possible, even with the hardware still holding the fracture together. As long as the fixation is stable, movement will help return the joint and adjacent muscles to a healthy state. Work on strength, balance, flexibility, and power.

Aging Feet

As you age, your foot usually gets a little bigger. Most people fail to realize this. You probably will need a larger shoe than you did in younger years. Moreover, as you get older your foot may be more prone to swelling.

If you are having a foot problem, buy a good running shoe. Wear shoes with laces that allow you to adjust the width, or obtain customized shoes or special soft inserts through a podiatrist.

Resources

If you have any foot problems, or are interested in prevention, it is well worth a visit to a podiatrist. Contact the American Podiatric Medical Association for the name of a podiatrist near you. The association, located in Bethesda, Maryland, can be contacted at 301-571-9200, or on the Internet at *www.apma.org*.

If you are actively involved in sports or regular exercise, I recommend seeing a sports podiatrist who belongs to the American Academy of Podiatric Sports Medicine. Contact the organization, in Rockville, Maryland (phone 800-438-3355, or on the Internet at *www.aapsm.org*).

Dr. Subotnick can be contacted by e-mail at *subots@aol.com*.

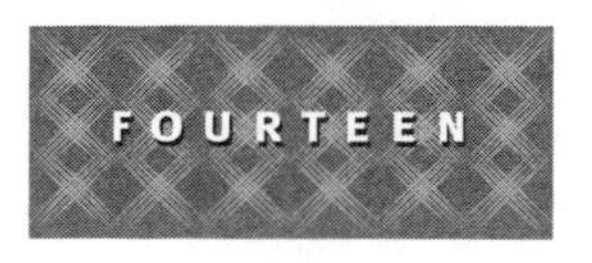

Sex and Your Joints

One of my most unusual cases involved an eighty-year-old male patient who was blind and diabetic, with congestive heart failure and generalized osteoarthritis. He was severely bent over because of the arthritis.

During one office visit he informed me he was having sex six times a day with his wife. I thought he was putting me on. But his wife, a woman of about sixty, was there and confirmed it. She joked and asked if there was some way I could slow down her husband's Olympian performance in bed.

I was astounded that anyone his age (or any age for that matter) and with his degree of infirmity could sustain such a level of sexual activity. Impotence often accompanies diabetes. Not in his case, however. This was his third wife. And he said he had been similarly potent for many years, despite poor health.

He said that not only did he crave and enjoy sex but the more sex he had the less pain he experienced from his arthritis.

Here was an individual with advanced osteoarthritis who used very little in the way of medication. He would take a couple of aspirins and that was it. Sex was his pain killer.

I asked his wife if he was waking her in the night in pain.

"He's waking me up," she said with a laugh, "but not for pain. For sex."

Sex as a painkiller?

Research indicates that certain substances called endorphins are released by the pituitary gland during orgasm. They are similar in chemical structure to morphine. Endorphin is a contraction for endogenously generated morphinelike substances. Besides an analgesic effect, endorphins also influence responses to stress, help determine mood, and stimulate the release of sex hormones. After sex, the release of endorphins promotes relaxation.

You have probably heard about endorphins. Strenuous exercise turns on your endorphins. They are often associated with a kind of euphoria—called "runner's high"—frequently experienced by recreational runners. Laughter also stimulates endorphin production.

Researchers say that orgasm, whether through sexual intercourse or masturbation, generates an endorphin response. Indeed, over the years, many patients have said they have experienced an average of about one to two hours of pain relief, sometimes significant, after orgasm. That's the equivalent of taking a morphine injection. My eighty-year-old patient experienced significant pain relief throughout the day from his multiple orgasms.

In *Natural Relief for Arthritis* (Emmaus, PA: Rodale Press, 1983), Carol Keough quoted a physician at the Cook County Hospital in Chicago who discovered this same pain-relieving effect accidentally among a number of handicapped patients with arthritis.

"They volunteered that sex helped them sometimes in striking ways," Wanda Sadoughi, M.D., commented. "They'd say, 'I was free of pain for several hours thereafter.'" Most of the patients were older and in some cases the arthritis was severe.

Orgasm also appears to trigger a generalized muscle relaxation that is probably a response of the hypothalamus, a center in the brain that regulates sex drive and also plays an important part in the emotions of pain and pleasure.

I suspected there was some kind of major muscle relaxation effect benefiting my eighty-year-old patient. This was at a time before we knew a good deal about endorphins. I have always considered that tight muscles produce stress on joints and reduce blood flow, thus creating irregular wear and tear on cartilage and lessened nourishment of the joints.

Years ago, in a clinical research setting, we tested the effect of orgasm on muscle tension through the use of electromyography, a technology that measures the condition of a muscle. We would place either needles or disk electrodes at the site of lumbar or hamstring muscles. The patient would then masturbate alone. Afterward, we would measure the muscle. We consistently found a profound level of muscle relaxation.

I am raising this subject because I believe that sexual intercourse provides both a preventive and therapeutic value in regard to osteoarthritis. Preventively, through muscle relaxation, stress release, and exercise. The exercise factor enters the picture because during intercourse the pelvis moves freely both in men and women. On a regular basis, the movement lubricates spinal joints, eases muscle tension, and reduces low-back stress.

As far as my amazing eighty-year-old patient was concerned, I didn't feel it was my place to ask him to refrain from having sex, as his wife wanted. But I did consult with the two of them and on a practical basis, I gave her some vaginal gels to help her with lubrication.

Sex, of course, offers many benefits for the body, soul, and mind. Arthritis prevention—and relief—may be another, as if added incentive was needed.

PART III

becoming an anti-arthritis warrior

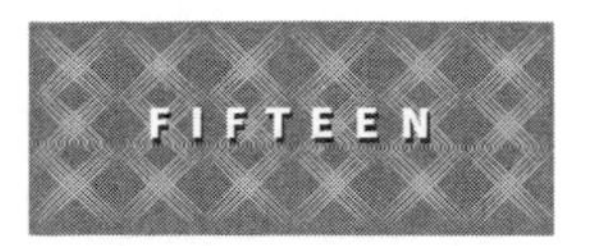

Putting It Together

Your task now is to become an anti-arthritis warrior and incorporate as many joint-friendly strategies as possible into your lifestyle. Some you'll find much easier to do than others. Some you already do. Some may not apply to you.

Don't take on too many changes at one time. Be practical.

And remember, that the investment you make in the health of your joints, pays off in dividends for the rest of your body. Eating better, keeping your weight down, exercising, taking nutritional supplements, and drinking plenty of water, for instance, help to keep all your parts working optimally.

Here, in review, are the main points of the ten steps to use as a quick guide to your personal prevention strategy. Put a check mark next to the points that most interest you and refer to the specific chapter for the details.

STEP 1. REDUCE REPETITIVE STRESS AND STRAIN ON MUSCLES AND JOINTS (CHAPTER 5)

- Be on the alert for chronic aches and strains that your job may be causing. You may need to rotate your task, modify your workstation, or even find an alternate job if you are developing symptoms. Bring the problem to the attention of your employer. Repetitive strain injury on the job is a major cause of soaring workers' compensation costs and lost productivity. Remember, such injury can create microtrauma in joints and adjacent soft tissues and lead to osteoarthritis in later years.

- See a qualified health professional such as an orthopedist, chiropractor, or podiatrist to determine if you have any structural risks for osteoarthritis. Even normal nonstressful activities can create degeneration over time in the presence of structural defects such as irregular cartilage surfaces, spinal misalignments, joint instability, or disturbed muscle nerve supply.
- Eliminate habits in your daily life that could be contributing to joint degeneration. The manner in which you hold the phone when talking, slouch while watching TV, and sit in a chair can be detrimental to your joint health.
- At the very first sign of chronic strain or pain, see a physician. Don't let it develop into something worse.

STEP 2. PROTECT YOUR JOINTS AFTER INJURY (CHAPTER 6)

- Injury to a joint is often a prelude to arthritis in the joint later in life.
- Take all proper precautions, including the use of safety equipment, in all your activities.
- There is much you can do to minimize the development of arthritis in joints after injury. Protective measures include acupuncture or massage to eliminate subsequent muscle spasm. Good nutrition, including wholesome food and supplements, speeds the healing process and brings blood-borne repair nutrients to injured sites.

STEP 3. EXERCISE (BUT DON'T ABUSE) YOUR JOINTS (CHAPTER 7)

- Neglecting exercise is not in your best interest. A sedentary lifestyle produces weak muscles and is widely thought to increase the odds of developing arthritis (and other health problems as well). Exercise makes you—and your joints—stronger and more flexible.
- See my Arthritis Prevention Exercise Program on page 90.
- Exercise daily, or at least every other day. If you haven't routinely exercised before, start modestly, and slowly increase your effort.
- Choose an activity you like. You are more likely to stick to it if you do. It doesn't have to be strenuous. Just regular.
- Consider a cross-training program that includes a variety of exercises. Cross-training helps prevents boredom.
- Incorporate light weight training into your exercise program to build denser bones and strengthen the muscles, ligaments, and tendons involved with joints.
- Avoid excess exercise that can raise the risk of injury and osteoarthritis.
- Undergo a physical examination with a sports medicine specialist, sports podiatrist, or other qualified medical professional before starting a regular exercise program. Check for, and correct, joint or other anatomical irregularities that might be aggravated by exercise.

STEP 4. EAT RIGHT AND TAKE A LOAD OFF YOUR JOINTS (CHAPTER 8)

- If you are too heavy, you're at higher risk for osteoarthritis. Losing weight cuts the risk.

- Diets generally don't work for the long term unless you exercise on a regular basis as well.
- Try my CICO (calories-in, calories-out) Diet, a simple dietary plan based on how many calories you eat and how many you burn off in activity. The process is helped by drinking a "vitamin C cocktail" before meals. Details of the diet begin on page 112.
- Chew your food well. It can actually help you lose weight!
- Eat food that is wholesome, and, if practical, organic. Processed and fast foods contain numerous chemical additives that are not in the best interest of your health. Such foods are often high in sugar and fat and deficient in important fiber and nutrients.

STEP 5. SUPPLEMENT YOUR JOINTS (CHAPTER 9)

- In a society habituated to processed and fast foods, nutritional supplements provide insurance against nutritional deficiencies.
- Alcohol, oral contraceptives, medication, environmental chemicals, and stress cause further nutrient deficiencies.
- Research shows that certain nutrients are vital for joint health. Supplements can help protect the joints and minimize or delay arthritic symptoms.
- See my Arthritis Prevention Supplement Program on page 168.

STEP 6. WATER YOUR THIRSTY JOINTS (CHAPTER 10)

- Drink plenty of water every day. Water is critical for the lubrication and shock-absorbing action of joints. See page 177 on how much to drink.
- Lack of sufficient water in the body may be a major underlying, and unrecognized, factor in joint degeneration and pain.

- Don't substitute sodas, coffee, and tea for water. In fact, they contain ingredients that may block the absorption of water or act like diuretics, that is, promote excretion of fluids from the body.

STEP 7. KEEP YOUR JOINTS FLEXIBLE WITH YOGA (CHAPTER 11)

- A few simple yoga postures can increase muscle tone and the flexibility and range of motion of joints. Research indicates that yoga generates beneficial mechanical pressures on joints.
- See the yoga program for arthritis prevention beginning on page 181. Practice the first five steps once or twice a day. If you have more time, do all seven steps.
- See the special yoga exercises on page 185 for hard-core computer users.

STEP 8. PROTECT YOUR HANDS (CHAPTER 12)

- The repetitive or forceful motions you perform with your hands can contribute to osteoarthritis.
- Are your hands "cool"? That could be a sign of susceptibility for osteoarthritis.
- See hand-saving tips on page 190, including fingerless gloves for "cool" hands and a simple massage technique.
- Long hours at the computer can strain and perhaps prematurely age your hands. Your joints could be affected over the long term unless you take some preventive action. See tips for computer users on page 193.

STEP 9. FOOT CARE—PREVENTING ARTHRITIS FROM THE GROUND UP (CHAPTER 13)

- Be shoe smart. Shoes can be a major cause of problems not just in the feet but in the knees and elsewhere in the body. Small shoes, dress shoes, high heels, are common troublemakers.
- The most protective footware? Running shoes and sandals with arches.
- See a podiatrist to determine the presence of any structural deformities or misalignments that could lead to irregular joint wear and osteoarthritis. The use of orthotic shoe inserts can help reduce structural problems.
- A podiatric evaluation for kids is a wise investment in their future foot health.
- Lose weight if you are too heavy. Excess weight contributes to osteoarthritis in the feet.

STEP 10. SEX AND YOUR JOINTS (CHAPTER 14)

- Add joint health to the list of benefits from orgasm.
- Sex produces substances in the body that relax the muscles, which, in turn, is good for the joints.
- There's also an exercise element to intercourse. That, too, is good for the joints.

above all, listen to your body

Along with all my other recommendations, I feel it important to repeat a commonsense theme I have mentioned previously in the book.

Remember the TV stockbrokerage commercial of a few years ago, "When E. F. Hutton talks, people listen"? What about when your body talks? Are you listening?

Minor aches and pains, for instance, are telling you something is wrong. They can, of course, be the result of a slight injury or they can be the prelude to a chronic condition, such as osteoarthritis.

In the early stages of arthritis, you may experience only sporadic joint discomfort or pain, which may be felt in association with activity. There is occasional stiffness and perhaps increasing difficulty carrying out routine daily tasks. Heed the message.

Experts such as Joseph A. Buckwalter, M.D., of the University of Iowa College of Medicine, and Debra Lappin, national chair of the Arthritis Foundation, point out that this is precisely the time, before more severe symptoms develop, to obtain a proper medical opinion.

Writing in the journal *Clinical Orthopaedics and Related Research* in March 2000, they note that in the early stages, there may be joint tenderness and slight restriction of joint motion. X rays may appear normal or show minimal loss of cartilage, small calcium deposits, and other changes in the bone tissue adjacent to the cartilage.

Now is the time, they urge, to take measures to slow down or prevent progression, such as avoiding repetitive impact and strain on affected joints, developing an exercise program, wearing impact-absorbing shoes, and, if indicated, losing weight.

I couldn't agree more. A problem may not start with outright pain, but rather a minor ache. If it becomes chronic, try to figure out what you are doing to cause it.

Take action immediately to prevent a minor problem from developing into severe pain later. That's good arthritis prevention. By listening to your body, you can take steps to perhaps eliminate the minor pain or keep it from escalating.

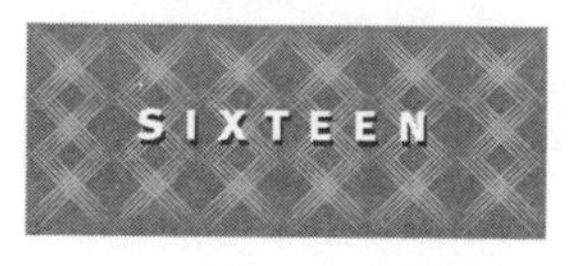

Doing the Extras—Acupuncture, Chiropractic, Massage, Rolfing

In this chapter I would like to mention a number of techniques available through the services of health professionals that can help prevent arthritis. They usually involve an out-of-pocket outlay on your part, but are definitely worth considering. Unfortunately, health insurance only tends to cover treatment for disease and not prevention of disease. It seems strange to even refer to it as health insurance. It should be called disease insurance. I have often wondered how much of the taxpayer's money we could save by covering proven prevention methods. Undoubtedly it would be a massive amount that could probably result in lowering taxes. But that's another issue.

At any rate, the extra preventive methods I would like to recommend are these:

- Acupuncture
- Chiropractic
- Massage
- Rolfing

acupuncture

With the opening of relations between the United States and China in the mid-1970s I went to the Orient as part of a delegation of physicians to observe the Chinese system of medical practice. The extensive and sophisticated use of acupuncture so impressed me that I subsequently studied the method and applied it for the benefit of my patients. In my experience, acupuncture has much to offer—both preventively and therapeutically.

Acupuncture is based on the Chinese concept of *qi* (pronounced "chee"), which roughly means energy, and its effect on how well the body functions.

During an acupuncture session, needles, with or without minute electrical currents attached, are inserted at specific locations in the body along meridians of energy. The needles push tissue out of the way with little, if any, discomfort. This is due in part to specially designed fine wire needles that have no edges.

The needles stimulate sensory nerve endings that send impulses up through the spinal cord to different areas of the brain, causing both local and central-acting effects. By stimulating these points, acupuncturists seek to restore normal energy flow and stimulate the body's ability to heal. The technique produces electrical and chemical changes. Blood vessels dilate. Nerve supply improves. Muscle spasm tends to relax. All this means more oxygen, nutrients, nerve stimulation, and reduced irregular pressures on joints. If you have pain, you experience relief. That's what my patients have consistently reported over the years.

During and after an acupuncture treatment that I know is going to affect a joint, I find that the joint is warmer to the touch than it was before treatment. This is a result of more blood and nerve supply reaching the area. I have also used medical measuring devices to corroborate these effects.

My positive clinical experience with acupuncture for arthritic patients prompted me many years ago to recommend periodic acupuncture "tune-ups" for patients as a preventive measure. Ideally, I suggest once a month, but even two or three times a year can be helpful. The tune-up involves one session and the use of thirty-two needle insertions from head to toe that increase blood flow throughout the body.

My observation is that the majority of patients who have followed a tune-up program over the years appear to be more flexible and have less symptoms from degenerative arthritis. I believe the treatments have also helped their general health.

Many of the modern medical studies on acupuncture have been done in China but have not been translated into English. Research in the West thus far has yielded "moderately strong evidence" and the validation of various expert committees. In 1997 a conference of experts sponsored by the National Institutes of Health endorsed the technique as a useful addition to treatment in a number of conditions, including osteoarthritis. This has led to increasing numbers of insurers covering acupuncture.

For pain relief, the number of acupuncture treatments will vary widely from person to person. For very severe pain or arthritic conditions, it could take up to twenty sessions, at the rate of two or three a week, before significant relief is felt. My advice to patients in these situations: Try another method if there is no relief by then. However, in many cases I have seen amazing relief after one or two sessions.

The veterinary experience with acupuncture is a powerful validation of this method. Animals, of course, are not subject to any placebo effect. They have no expectations or beliefs in a treatment method that could translate into relief. Veterinarians say it works for many acute and chronic disorders, and pain conditions, in addition to serving as an effective prevention and health-maintenance technique. Some veterinarians believe acupuncture is the best pain reliever of all the alternative therapies, especially for chronic pain and relief of musculoskeletal symptoms from arthritis, disk disorders, lameness, and stiff backs.

Resources

For more information on acupuncture, including referrals, schools of acupuncture, licensing criteria, and articles on specific treatments, contact the American Association of Oriental Medicine, in Catasauqua, Pennsylvania (phone: 888-500-7999; on the Internet at *www.aaom.org*).

chiropractic

There is not a great deal of scientific data on the incidence of osteoarthritis of the spine. What little research is available suggests strongly that the condition is common. My clinical experience tells me this is indeed so. I have treated numerous patients over the years for pain associated with degeneration of both the spinal disks and the vertebral joints.

I have referred patients for many years to chiropractors, health professionals who use manipulative techniques to address misalignments in the spine and other joints throughout the body. There is a large body of research on these techniques, in particular demonstrating effectiveness for acute and chronic low-back and neck pain.

I believe that chiropractic also has value in the prevention and treatment of osteoarthritis. For that reason I recommend that patients obtain a periodic chiropractic evaluation, whether they have symptoms or not.

Structure affects function, and structural misalignments in the spine can have numerous impacts of bodily function. A misalignment means that a bone or joint is not in its normal position. It can be caused by trauma at birth, injury, the overuse of one side of the body, poor posture, weaknesses in the spine, and discrepancies in leg length (one leg is longer than the other).

A "pot belly," common in our overeating and underexercising society, is another potential cause for misalignment. The excess abdominal weight creates a marked increase in the curvature of the lumbar (low-back) spine. The resultant stress can upset joint and soft-tissue alignments locally as well as elsewhere in the spine, leading to degenerative disk and vertebral changes.

A misalignment can impinge on a nerve that radiates from the spinal column. This can cause pain, loss of bodily function associated with the particular nerve, and reduced energy. A misaligned joint can create a loss of range of motion and with that a reduction in microcirculation. The affected site becomes cut off from normal nerve and nutrient supply. Result: degeneration and the development of the arthritic process.

Moreover, misalignments in the bony structures, or even in the surrounding soft tissues such as muscles, tendons, and ligaments, can create stress shears, that is, irregular pressures on joints. These also create a degenerative scenario involving blood-vessel changes, calcium deposition, and destruction of cartilage.

Misalignment in the spine can occur in one spot or at multiple locations from the neck down to the lower part of the back.

You need a proper evaluation to determine the presence of a misalignment that may be causing pain, malfunction, or otherwise silently setting the stage for arthritic problems later in life. Medical doctors are not trained to do that. Chiropractors and osteopathic physicians are. They have been specially trained to evaluate and address misalignments by corrective manipulations.

These "adjustments" are performed to help restore normal motion to affected joints. And this, in turn, improves mechanical and nerve function, relaxes tight muscles, and reopens the flow of nutrients, nerve supply, and endorphins, the body's own natural pain killers. In this way, joint degeneration may be prevented or stopped.

A preventive chiropractic checkup once a year is a good idea. If an evaluation reveals an underlying joint problem, consider having it corrected. The earlier you spot and correct a misalignment the less chance of it leading to arthritic changes. In addition to manipulative techniques, many chiropractors also apply a variety of other methods such as nutrition, exercise, and electrical muscle stimulation to improve joint health.

I should say, however, that I do not believe in chiropractic treatments two or three times a week that go on indefinitely. Overmanipulation can create laxity of tissue and loose ligaments.

Joint evaluations may also be performed by osteopaths, physicians who receive a standard medical education along with extra training in spinal health. However, most manipulations these days are performed by chiropractors.

Spinal evaluations and the use of appropriate manipulation techniques represent a major physical medicine tool for spinal integrity that is overlooked in both the prevention and treatment of osteoarthritis.

Resources

If you need help finding a chiropractor in your area, contact the American Chiropractic Association in Arlington, Virginia (phone: 800-986-4638; on the Internet at *www.amerchiro.org/*).

massage

Many years ago, a Finnish man opened a massage business near my pain clinic in North Hollywood. I started going there regularly in an effort to rid my body of accumulated stresses from a busy medical practice. I felt so good from the experience that I began recommending that patients try it as well. One of them was a middle-aged aircraft mechanic who developed early osteoarthritis in the shoulders as a result of repetitive strain injury. His job required working intensely for long periods of time with his arms overhead. A series of massages, he reported, had given him considerably more mobility and reduced the pain.

At the time I didn't know exactly how or if massage could specifically help osteoarthritis, but I did hear from quite a few patients with arthritis that they consistently felt better after massage treatment.

I found many answers to my curiosity about massage after I became interested in Chinese medicine. When most people think about Chinese medicine, acupuncture and Chinese herbs come to mind. But there is another major aspect to their great inventory of healing knowledge: massage. I was quite surprised to learn that the Chinese have always put great stock in massage. They, as well as the Indians, have an elaborate system of massage that dates back to very ancient texts. Neither, however, can lay claim to the discovery of massage, probably one of the oldest healing methods known to mankind. Did it start with some cave dweller eons ago who found that rubbing a bruised muscle made it feel better?

As I learned more and heard continuing feedback from patients, I became increasingly impressed with massage. I eventually incorporated massage therapy into my pain practice. I found that patients with arthritis achieved a great deal of benefit from regular massage and seemed to achieve a level of help similar to that obtained from acupuncture and herbs.

Massage is quite a universal practice and involves numerous types of techniques. I learned this from much traveling abroad. I have probably had massages in fifty countries, including China, Norway, India, Russia, Kenya, and Tanzania.

Today, a growing volume of research has accumulated validating the benefits of massage therapy for a wide range of medical conditions, including arthritis, pain, and rehabilitation from injury. Many physicians prescribe massage as a standard part of treatment programs, and hospitals are increasingly bringing massage therapists on staff.

Massage, of course, makes you feel good. It does that, according to the American Massage Therapy Association, by reducing the heart rate and blood pressure, increasing blood circulation and lymph flow, relaxing muscles, alleviating muscle spasm, improving range of motion, and boosting endorphins and serotonin, chemicals in the body related to feeling good and feeling calm.

I have always been fascinated by the effect of massage on lymph.

Based on local massage traditions that go back centuries, all masseuses believe that their methods rid the body of toxins. I don't dispute this. Thus massage may act in preventing toxins from ending up in joint or adjacent tissues. Such toxins could be involved in some way in the arthritic process.

Massage stimulates lymph circulation and drainage of poisons from the body. This is a major element of the body's waste-removal and immune system that American medicine tends to neglect. We fail to realize that one of the reasons joints swell is lymphostasis. The lymph just isn't moving. I recall the case of a female patient who arrived in my office one day with a hugely swollen and painful arthritic knee. The tissue was soft on palpation. I suspected the grossly abnormal swelling was from lymphostasis. I treated her with massage and the next day she called to say the swelling, and much of the pain, had disappeared.

If there is a toxic element to osteoarthritis, then massage offers a major preventive and therapeutic benefit by promoting the normal movement and drainage of lymph through the body. Exercise, of course, is a primary stimulator of lymph flow, as well as blood flow.

Some patients, no matter how much I have nagged them, never do any exercise or other form of relaxation. For such people, massage is ideal. Somebody can do it for them. A professional massage is the best, of course. But if you don't want to spend the money, you can practice some self-massage yourself (see the box below) or have your wife, husband, boyfriend, or girlfriend perform the massage.

Simple Self-Massage

Depending on how much time you have, perform a short and simple daily massage on the parts of the body you use the most. You will notice as you perform the massage that the area warms up. This is a result of the increased blood flow.

(continued on next page)

(continued from previous page)

If it is not unduly messy for you, you might like to use a bit of sesame or almond oil as you work the soft tissue. Sesame oil is used in Indian massage and is said to help remove toxins from the tissue.

If you work a lot with your hands, such as at the computer, refer to chapter 12 for a simple massage to your hands and forearms you can do whenever you take a break.

If you feel tension building up in your neck at the end of a workday, give it a little tender loving care. With the fingertips of both hands, press the flesh along the spine. Move with firm pressure up and down your neck. Don't press so hard that it is painful. Just good, firm pressure.

A daily self-massage to the bottoms of the feet has bodywide benefits. The soles contain a concentration of acupuncture points. You are helping your feet and energizing the entire body as well. Also tug on the toes and perform a squeezing action from your toe tips up to your calves. This stimulates blood and lymph flow.

Patients have always asked me which massage is the best. I believe that the best massage is the one that makes you feel the best, and this varies from person to person. You need to experiment. Try a variety of massages and see which one you like. Some people respond to shiatsu, others to Swedish massage, or to deep-tissue massage. There is a marvelous head-to-foot massage from India, *abyanga,* in which you are massaged with sesame oil. This massage is available in clinics specializing in Ayurveda, the traditional health system of India.

Resources

To find a qualified massage therapist near you, contact the American Massage Therapy Association in Evanston, Illinois (phone: 888-843-2682; on the Internet at *www.amtamassage.org*).

rolfing

Today, at age seventy-five, I stand as tall as I did when I was in high school. That is quite unusual. One of the proven indicators for health in going the distance is having the same height and weight you had as a senior in high school. Happily, I have both of them. I attribute it, among other things, to Rolfing.

Rolfing, in case you haven't heard the term, is an extremely effective system of body work developed decades ago by Dr. Ida Rolf, a biochemist at the Rockefeller Institute. The method involves a series of ten sessions administered by a certified Rolfer who manually works the soft tissue of the body from head to toe in order to reintroduce structural integration that has been lost over time.

People seek out Rolfers to ease pain and chronic stress, or, in the case of athletes, to improve performance. Research shows that Rolfing generates more effective use of the muscles, creates a better pattern of movement, reduces chronic stress and pain and undesirable changes in body mechanics.

> *This is the gospel of Rolfing: When the body gets working appropriately, the force of gravity can flow through. Then, spontaneously, the body heals itself.*
>
> **IDA P. ROLF**

I have found that the effect of Rolfing is most pronounced on the elongation of the spine and greatly aids joint function. The postural changes associated with aging and arthritis are deterred.

I have referred many patients to Benjamin Shield, Ph.D., a skilled Rolfer in West Los Angeles.

"Just as a chiropractor works with the hard, bony tissue, Rolfers normalize the skeletal structure and joint mechanics by manipulating the soft tissue," says Shield. "We work with the myofascia that consists of the body's muscles, tendons, ligaments, and fascia."

Structural misalignments and compensations, postural habits, overuses, emotional holding patterns, and injuries to the soft tissue create undue tension and stress on the joints. "This impairment of joint function," he adds, "can create inflammation, pain, and accelerated wear and tear of the joints. When this happens, the body reacts by tightening the soft tissue around the joint, which causes more compression, improper joint mechanics, pain, and joint degeneration. This causes even more tightening around the joint and it becomes a vicious cycle resulting in osteoarthritis."

We tend not to hear much about fascia, a network of connective tissue that provides support throughout the body. Fascia envelopes every aspect of our anatomy: the muscles, bones, vital organs, and even the microscopic structures within our cells.

Rolfers manipulate the fascia and other soft tissue to lengthen what has become tight, to relieve adhesions, and to bring the body's structure back to balance. Using manual techniques with various degrees of pressure, from fine and gentle to very firm, they progress from area to area, relieving abnormal pressures and unhealthy patterns of soft-tissue function throughout the body. Each pattern is unique to every individual, so each case is treated differently.

I am a great admirer of both massage and Rolfing. Many people confuse the two. There are important differences. "The purpose of massage is to relax the individual, stretch tight muscles, detoxify, and stimulate various body systems," explains Shield. "These benefits are also a by-product of Rolfing. However, the intention of Rolfing is to change and integrate the structure in such a way that there is a visible and perceptual change with each session. We progressively bring the person closer to balance, improved function, greater freedom of motion, and less pain with each treatment."

The typical Rolfing series of ten treatments usually involves once-a-week sessions. Each session lasts about an hour to an hour and a half. A Rolfer may also work "outside the series" to treat a particular condition.

Many physicians familiar with Rolfing prescribe a treatment series for patients with painful musculoskeletal problems such as arthritis. Health insurance often covers the treatment if a doctor prescribes it. Prevention, however, may be a different story. You probably will have to pay for the expense of treatments yourself, which typically runs around $100 per session.

Do you need follow-up treatment after a typical series of ten sessions? Sometimes symptoms will return and individuals will want a Rolfing "tune-up." In many other cases, people feel so good from their Rolfing experience that they come back for more advanced treatments in an attempt to keep feeling better.

Rolfing is not a cure for arthritis. Nor does it necessarily cause the joints to rebuild and undo the wear and tear already done. However, it creates a healthier environment around the joint and improves function.

"I see people with various degrees of osteoarthritis involving a few or many joints," says Shield. "I regularly work on people with arthritis of the spine, shoulder, elbow, knee, jaw, and hips."

Shield, who has been practicing for eighteen years, finds that Rolfing is extremely effective to reduce pain and improve range of motion.

"In some cases we can give long-term relief to someone with arthritis," he says. "In other cases, where the arthritis is very severe, the improvement may be moderate. My experience, based on more than 25,000 treatments, is that there is no question that Rolfing improves the anatomy and functioning of the joints and soft tissue. It slows down the arthritic process. It allows people to be more active, with less discomfort and more choices in their lives."

Rolfers don't just work the area of an affected joint. They work on the whole body in an attempt to normalize the entire structure and restore healthy patterns of functioning to the soft tissue.

"If we just worked on a single area, the misaligned patterns that exist throughout the rest of the body would most likely recreate the old unhealthy pattern," Shield says. "We look to change and normalize the whole structure and bring it to balance. We are not looking for short-term fixes."

In a Discovery Health Channel segment on Rolfing aired in 2000, one of Shield's patients was filmed before, during, and after treatment. The patient was Lonnie Grant, fifty-one, a Los Angeles–area personal trainer and martial artist, who suffers from severe osteoarthritis in his shoulders. As Grant tells it, "I have a body like a machine with some parts now in disrepair from years of contact sports, weight training, and overtraining."

Severe shoulder pain plus decreasing range of motion prompted Grant to undergo shoulder surgery. However, the procedure did not provide any significant improvement in range of motion and relief of pain.

"That's because the same underlying soft-tissue conditions existed after surgery as before," says Shield.

A discouraged Grant sought out alternative methods and discovered Rolfing. He was now taking two Advils after heavy workouts and particularly following one-on-one martial arts classes where he had to make many quick moves. "I needed that in order to reduce the pain and be able to sleep," he says.

Since Rolfing, Grant says, he has had much less pain and hasn't had to resort to medication as often.

Is Rolfing for arthritis prevention worth the money? If you have the money, I say do it. Car owners know that you have to bring in a vehicle for periodic maintenance and preventive care. You want your car aligned properly and the parts working with each other in good order. Rolfing does just that for the body. It keeps the joints from becoming compressed as a result of undesirable rotational and compensational patterns caused by injuries, posture, and life's activities. The effect is to prolong the healthy and efficient biomechanics of the joints. Take it from a doctor who has been treating painful and damaged joints for a half-century. Rolfing is a great benefit. This is real preventive medicine—without the medicine. If you feel discomfort or achiness in any of your joints, run, don't walk to your nearest Rolfer. And even if you don't feel any discomfort, think prevention.

Resources

For those interested in more details, see Ida P. Rolf's book *Rolfing* (Rochester, VT: Healing Arts Press, 1989).

To find a Rolfer near you, contact the Rolf Institute in Boulder, Colorado (phone: 800-530-8875; or on the Internet at *www.rolf.org*).

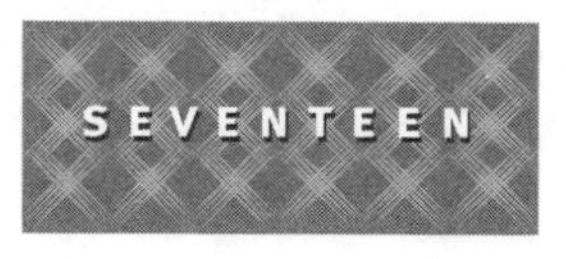

If You Already Have Arthritis: Relieving Symptoms and Preventing Them from Getting Worse*

There is no single solution for the symptoms of osteoarthritis. Once you have the condition, you have it. Although we are making huge advances in medical science, we don't yet have a cure for osteoarthritis. Most of the time, a physician will recommend pain medication, or, if necessary, joint replacement. These may indeed be required in many cases, but there are many other options at your disposal that will certainly decrease pain, improve stiffness and range of motion, and, in general, produce overall relief. You can become an anti-arthritis warrior even if you have the condition. You *can* take action to lessen your symptoms and limitations.

As you step up the battle against arthritis, just remember that you are an individual and that one particular weapon may work better for you than the next person, depending on the severity and location of your arthritis.

The options include exercise, diet, supplements, yoga, massage, and the use of hot tubs. All the ideas described in Part Two may also be quite effective for relief as well.

---

* See also the discussions of acupuncture, chiropractic, massage, and Rolfing in chapter 16.

Losing weight if you are overweight, starting an exercise program, eating right and taking certain supplements, and drinking plenty of water are going to improve symptoms. I can't tell you which combination of recommendations is better than another. Only you can tell. And not every recommendation may apply to your situation. My advice is to follow the appropriate recommendations in a comfortable way and determine what works best for you. One approach may be the key to relief. Adding other measures may provide smaller, but nevertheless welcome benefits.

exercise (See chapter 7 on exercise.)

In the past, exercise was discouraged for patients with arthritis. The fear was that vigorous motion could damage fragile arthritic joints. Instead, rest and decreased joint use were usually prescribed as a means to improve painful joints.

We now have a different attitude toward exercise. Arthritis patients frequently have decreased physical fitness, as measured by reduced range of motion, stability of joints, muscle weakness, and poor aerobic capacity. They have more pain and stiffness. These negative developments result from the underlying disease and all its consequences, including the side effects of medication and most certainly decreased physical activity. A direct causal relationship has not been demonstrated, but poor physical fitness is associated with higher levels of pain and disability in arthritis patients.

For all these reasons, we now regard exercise as safe and beneficial for arthritics. The aim is to improve fitness, keep joints flexible, and improve muscle strength, thereby reducing pain, stiffness, and disability.

And for arthritics who may be depressed because of their illness, exercise also serves to uplift the mood. Duke University researchers recently reported that exercise appeared to be superior even to Zoloft, one of the mainstream medical drugs, in reducing major depression and keeping the condition from returning.

The U.S. Surgeon General recommends getting thirty minutes of moderate activity daily. That's a wonderful goal to put your sights on. But if you can't quite manage to do that much, please do whatever you can on a regular basis. It is so beneficial.

Recent studies indicate that important health gains can be achieved just with a relatively modest effort. As M. T. Galloway and Peter Jokl of Yale commented in a medical paper on success aging, "the greatest benefit is seen when one goes from doing nothing to doing something."

A regular program of doing something not only helps your joints and alleviates pain, but will help your heart, enhance weight loss if you are too heavy, and reduce stress. In my experience of treating thousands of patients with osteoarthritis over the years, I have found that those who exercise have invariably felt better than those who have not. Among other things, they were usually able to reduce their intake of pain medication, making them less susceptible to side effects.

And last, but certainly not least, people who exercise regularly live longer and are healthier than sedentary individuals.

But exercise is like medicine. You have to continue doing it, just as you have to continue taking the medicine. Otherwise the benefits disappear. This was made very clear in an American-Canadian study led by Theresa Sullivan, M.A., of the University of Manitoba. Initially, the researchers found that an eight-week program of supervised fitness walking, plus patient education, generated meaningful improvement in functional status for individuals with knee osteoarthritis. In that short period of time, the participants in the study were able to stretch out their walking distance by 18 percent without any aggravation of pain or need for more medication. A year later the researchers contacted many of the patients to see if they were still walking on their own. The findings were disappointing. Most had stopped and had lost their conditioning benefits.

First and foremost, see your physician before starting any exercise program. If your physician can't help you with specific recommendations, he or she can likely refer you to a qualified physical therapist, chiropractor, osteopath, or sports medicine or rehabilitation specialist. This is particularly important if you have moderate to severe arthritis of the weight-bearing joints.

Improper exercising, or the presence of unstable joints, structural abnormalities, or muscle weakness can exacerbate arthritis. The benefits of exercise are huge, even for people with advanced arthritis, so seek out an expert to guide you. It is better to be safe than sorry. Don't consult personal trainers in health spas for exercise advice if you have arthritis. Although some may be knowledgeable, in general they don't have the background to instruct you in a way that carefully protects and strengthens arthritic joints.

Varying the type of exercise helps many people stick to the exercise habit. If you have sore knees, for instance, a good alternative is cycling outdoors or riding an indoor stationary bike.

For Individuals with Mobility Limitations

Let your chair serve as a launch pad to greater activity. Some people who exercise in chairs can later move on to other activities. Simple exercises done right in the chair can stimulate the heart, lungs, and muscles. A pedal machine in front of a chair also offers good aerobic exercise.

Resources

Get Fit While You Sit: Easy Workouts from Your Chair, by Charlene Torkelson (Alameda, CA: Hunter House, 1999).

How to Begin an Exercise Session

Arthritics generally need to take more time to warm up. There are a number of reasons for this. One is that they often have muscle spasm, and you don't want to exercise against tight muscles. So take a bit of time to loosen and stretch the muscles. You may also want to massage the muscles that are more likely to bother you.

All this will also help to lubricate and loosen joints. In addition, warming up will increase blood flow to the body parts that may have some circulatory impairment because of the arthritis.

I suggest at least ten minutes for a good warm-up.

How to Tell If You Are Doing Too Much

There's a simple formula. You overdid it if you exercise today and tomorrow you awaken with more discomfort and pain than you had today. That's what I tell my patients. You cannot evaluate your exercise tolerance based on how you feel immediately afterward. Usually you will feel better right after exercising, even if you have severe arthritis. But the key is how you feel the day after. Cut back some on the exercise the next time out if you feel worse.

Exercise for Arthritis of the Hands

I recommend Play-Doh, the soft, pliable, and colorful modeling compound that kids love to roll up into balls, snakes, or other creations.

For arthritis of the hands, roll up a piece into a ball that fits comfortably in the hand. Then repeatedly squeeze the ball and relax the hand. Squeeze and relax. Alternate hands.

As a general rule, use a lotion or Vaseline to lubricate the hands. Soft skin over arthritic joints promotes better range of motion.

Exercise for Arthritis of the Feet

I recommend taking a small rolling pin and using it to massage the bottom of the feet. One foot at a time, please, unless you are sitting in a chair. Repeatedly move the feet back and forth over the pin.

The best exercise is walking. I have covered that in detail in chapter 7.

See a podiatrist for an evaluation. Refer to chapter 13 on foot care.

Exercise for Arthritis of the Knees

- Be sure to strengthen the quadriceps muscle (the big muscle in the front of the thighs). Weak "quads" cause problems in the knees. Strong "quads" provide protection. Refer to the section on weight training in chapter 7 on how to build up this important muscle.

- You also want to strengthen the knee muscles to act as shock absorbers for the joint. The knee should be conditioned to the point where it can be exercised normally. One simple way to do it is with an isometric exercise in which you alternately tighten and relax the muscles around the kneecap. Isometrics involves contracting muscles while the joint stays in one position. In this case, lie on your back and extend your legs. Tighten the knee muscles to a count of 1-100, 2-100, 3-100, 4-100, 5-100. Then relax for a count of 1-100, 2-100. As you become stronger, you can sustain the contraction for longer counts, and you may notice less pain or a greater sense of comfort during walking or other activities. If both knees are affected, do the exercise first with one knee and then the other.

- Safe, weight-bearing exercise should involve a full range of motion for your legs. Studies have found that patients with osteoarthritis of the knees can tolerate walking.

- If you choose to walk for exercise, your safest surfaces are level grass or dirt (be very sure there are no holes), or a synthetic running track (known as a tartan track), if one is located nearby. Try to avoid pavement. Reduce your speed if you feel your knees are being irritated. Long-term aerobic walking, along with a weight-training program has been found effective in significantly improving postural stability and balance among older individuals with arthritic knees. Difficulty with balance, as a result of arthritis or other disorders, can increase the risk of falls and injury to the hips and other joints.

- If you develop worse knee pain and swelling after a short walk, see a specialist to discuss alternative exercises.
- Swimming and cycling are good alternative exercises. In general, swimming is particularly helpful for the pain and stiffness of lower back problems and arthritis of the knees.
- Avoid high impact activities. Don't overstress your knees.
- Avoid activities such as golf and tennis, which generate potentially harmful torsional forces on the knees.
- Be sure to wear good shoes, with solid soles and heels. See chapter 13 on foot care.
- Have your feet evaluated by a podiatrist. You may have a deviation in your foot structure that is putting extra pressure on a particular part of the knee joint. Heel wedges or orthotics can often correct the problem.
- Avoid standing for long periods of time. Take the load off your knees with frequent rests.
- Keep bending or squatting to a minimum.
- If possible, elevate the level of beds, chairs, and toilets to minimize the degree of knee bending.
- Avoid stairs. If you can't, take them slowly.

arthritis, pain, and food (See chapter 8 on diet and weight.)

We know that overweight people are at higher risk for arthritis, and research is beginning to show that weight reduction, even slight, can help relieve symptoms for those who have arthritis of the weight-bearing joints.

My clinical experience has shown that the combination of diet with exercise, as I described in chapter 8, can indeed be helpful for relief.

I have also learned from my patients that a diet high in sugar, and primarily white sugar, can contribute to pain. I first made the connection with arthritic patients years ago. The more sugar they ate, the more pain they had. When they cut down on the sugar they had less pain. I have observed this phenomenon repeatedly, and many physicians at pain conferences have told me they have also noticed this effect.

I routinely advise arthritic patients to cut out sugar as much as possible. This means not only the sugar you put in your cereal, coffee, or tea, but also the massive amounts hidden in food items such as soda, chocolate cake, chocolate chip cookies, and ice cream.

Sugar interferes with calcium's role in electrochemical transmissions in the body, causing nerves to become irritated.

Alcoholic beverages often worsen pain. Sometimes small amounts of alcohol, which relax a patient, seem to be helpful, but spirits should be avoided and especially if you have chronic pain.

Fried or fatty foods can also aggravate a chronic pain condition. The effects of such foods will not be felt until forty-five minutes or an hour after eating. Fatty meals generate substances called chylomicrons. They are fatty droplets that appear in the blood. When they enter small capillaries they tend to decrease blood flow. The result is reduced oxygen and nutrients to sensitive tissues such as arthritic joints.

nutritional supplements for relief (See chapter 9 on nutritional supplements.)

There's no supplement, or combination of supplements, created on this planet that magically restores arthritic joints to a pre-arthritic status. Supplements can't cure osteoarthritis. But the very good news, if you have arthritis, is that certain supplements can substantially reduce symptoms and deter progression of the disease.

For people on medication, a supplement program is additionally important because some medical drugs cause nutritional deficiencies.

Keep in mind also that each of us is a unique individual with different genetic makeup, size, hormonal activity, tolerances, energy, resistance, and levels of health or illness. Even if two people have the same severity of osteoarthritis in the same joint, each brings into play a different set of strengths and weaknesses with which to counteract the condition. Thus, because we are so different, our bodies respond somewhat differently to medication. One aspirin may work to relieve your joint pain in the knee but a sibling with similar pain may need more. The same concept holds true for natural remedies and nutritional supplements.

A basic rule of thumb is to take the least possible amount that gives you the benefit you desire. And because we are not talking cure, you generally experience relief for as long as you use supplements. If you discontinue supplements, the benefits may cease rapidly or gradually.

Following are a selection of nutritional supplements that offer benefits. Substances such as glucosamine and chondroitin sulfate are known to be chondroprotective, that is, appear to stop progression as well as reduce symptoms. MSM, which reduces symptoms, may also be chondroprotective. Other individual supplements have not been proven to stop progression, but help reduce symptoms.

You may have to experiment with different combinations or products to find one that works best for you. And remember that nutritional supplements are not drugs. They go to work in your body immediately but you won't feel the results in a half-hour as you would with a drug. Symptom relief usually takes days, weeks, or even months, depending on the severity of the condition. Please be patient. Your patience will pay off.

If you are taking prescription medicine for your condition, you may find that the supplements provide substantial relief and that you don't require as much medication. However, do not reduce the medication without speaking to your doctor. In any case, consult with your doctor before you start a supplement program.

Supplements to Reduce Symptoms

Use supplements on a *daily basis*. Dosages shown here are for daily use.

If any particular supplement produces discomfort, reduce the dosage or stop taking it.

Purchase the nearest potency if you cannot find the supplement at the same strength that I recommend.

In general, you can find higher-quality and more advanced supplements in health-food stores.

STEP 1

Start the following supplements at the same time:

- A multivitamin and -mineral formula. Some of the leading manufacturers make products that are age or gender specific and that also contain antioxidants and nutraceuticals.
- Vitamin C—at least 1,000 milligrams.
- Glucosamine—1,500 milligrams, usually taken in three divided doses of 500 milligrams each.
- Chondroitin sulfate—1,200 milligrams, taken as 400 milligrams three times a day.
- MSM—3,000 to 8,000 milligrams.

The marketplace contains many formulas for joint health with different combinations of ingredients. Among the most popular and effective ingredients are glucosamine, chondroitin, and MSM. Be sure, however, to read the warnings in chapter 9 about glucosamine and chondroitin products. If you don't feel any relief from a combination within a few weeks, add extra MSM and increase the

(continued on next page)

(continued from previous page)

amount slowly (see the MSM section in chapter 9 for details). You can also try another combination formula if the first one doesn't help.

All multivitamin and mineral formulas contain some vitamin C, but may not have as much as I recommend. If the amount is less than 1,000 milligrams, take an extra vitamin C supplement. A multi will often contain 400 IUs of vitamin D. But if you are elderly and live in a northern climate, consider taking additional D during the winter months.

Step 2

Start the following supplements in any order at one-week intervals.

- Vitamin E—400 to 800 IUs
- Niacinamide—500 milligrams three or four times a day
- Vitamin B6—100 to 200 milligrams
- Omega-3 fatty acids—2 to 3 grams
- Boron—up to 9 milligrams daily
- Sam-e—at least 200 milligrams
- Magnesium—100 milligrams to start, then go up to 300 to 400 milligrams in divided daily doses

Your multivitamin and -mineral formula will contain some of these elements but probably not as much as I have recommended.

yoga therapy (See chapter 11 on yoga.)

Yoga contributes in a major way to the healing force within each of us. According to the American Yoga Association, it provides a gentle, safe, methodical exercise and relaxation program that eases the discomforts of chronic arthritis. The practice "encourages you to keep moving gently . . . in order to maintain muscle tone, good circulation, and joint flexibility," the association says. "Arthritis does not have to be a disability. By practicing a few gentle exercises, breathing, and meditation every day, you can reduce pain, build your strength, and maintain your daily activities with health and renewed energy."

Research has begun to confirm what practitioners of yoga have long known, that this ancient practice can benefit arthritic patients. In a 1994 study published in the *Journal of Rheumatology,* researchers described significant improvement from yoga for pain, tenderness, and range of motion among patients with osteoarthritis in the hands.

In a 1983–1984 survey of individuals suffering from a variety of ailments and who were prescribed yoga as an alternative therapy, 90 percent of 589 arthritis patients reported benefits from the practice. The survey was conducted by the Yoga Biomedical Trust in England.

There are many books about the therapeutic benefits of yoga, and in them are chapters or references to arthritis. While these can often be helpful, best results are usually obtained from an individualized program. In the beginning some patients may only be able to do minimal limb movements. Some may be in such pain that they can only start with a breathing exercise (see chapter 11). Remember that breathing alone moves the body, and even if that's all that can be done, the breathing exercise turns on the healing mode and has surprisingly beneficial effects.

I strongly recommend working with a knowledgeable physician or a specially trained expert in yoga therapy (see resources below) who can develop a customized program for you and oversee your progress. It's well worth the money.

Larry Payne, Ph.D., author of *Yoga for Dummies,* points out that patients should seek out a yoga therapist just as they would seek out a specialist for any medical condition. "A skilled professional takes into account your condition, your age, and your lifestyle to create a routine that will be the most effective," he says.

Payne has done this for many individuals with back pain and arthritis over the years, helping them to relieve pain and reestablish flexibility in arthritic joints.

One of his pupils is Ingrid Kelsey, a seventy-seven-year-old retired legal administrator in Malibu, California, with severe lumbar osteoarthritis. Until she started yoga more than five years ago, she had been on strong pain medication.

Now, as she tells it, "I have pain only occasionally during the night and in the morning. I can usually manage it by doing a few yoga exercises."

Ingrid attends classes twice a week and practices yoga stretches on a daily basis after arising in the morning.

"There was a gradual reduction in the pain after I began practicing yoga," she says. "Only now and then do I need to take an Advil for the pain. Yoga has made a big difference for me."

Ingrid also reports that increasing stiffness in her lower back has accompanied the progress of her arthritis. However, she says, "yoga always removes it quickly."

Taking action: Many people with arthritis may be able to perform on their own the first five steps of Payne's yoga arthritis-prevention program (again, refer back to chapter 11). Do them once or twice a day. Try to work your way slowly up to a full half-hour. If you have more time, try to do the sixth and seventh steps as well.

"Challenge but don't strain the body," says Payne. And if you have any doubts, see a yoga therapist.

RESOURCES

To find a nearby yoga therapist, contact the International Association of Yoga Therapists in Lower Lake, California (phone: 707-928-9898; on the Internet at *www.yrec.org*). You can also refer to the popular periodical *The Yoga Journal* available at many bookstores, newsstands and health-food stores.

Two articles on arthritis, written by Mary Schatz, M.D., have appeared in the journal over the years, and reprints can be obtained from the Yoga Research and Education Center (same phone number as above). The articles are entitled "Yoga for Arthritis," November/December 1997, and "Yoga Relief for Arthritis," May/June 1985.

Book resources include *Yoga for Dummies* (Foster City, CA: IDG Books Worldwide, 1999), by Georg Feuerstein and Larry Payne; *Yoga for Common Ailments* (New York: Simon & Schuster, 1990), by R. Monro, R. Nagarathna, and H. R. Nagendra; *Yoga for Wellness: Healing with the Timeless Teachings of Viniyoga* (New York: Penguin/Arkana, 1999), by Gary Kraftsow; and *The American Yoga Association Wellness Book* (New York: Kensington Books, 1996), by Alice Christensen.

osteomassage (self-massage)

In chapter 16, I explained how massage helps prevent or treat arthritis by improving blood and lymph movement, relaxing tight muscles, enhancing the range of motion, and elevating compounds in the body, such as endorphins, that reduce pain and make you feel better.

You might also like to try a method of massage on your own or with the help of a spouse or friend. It is called osteomassage.

In 1973 I began developing and reporting on a pain-relief technique called osteopuncture that involved stimulation of the periosteum—the thin covering of the surface of bone. The method is performed by a physician who inserts small needles into this covering tissue at various points throughout the body. Numerous doctors around the world have used osteopuncture to treat many thousands of patients.

Osteomassage is an outgrowth of this work, a logical extension that requires only the fingertips to stimulate the covering of the bone with a simple circular motion. It is something you can do by yourself for many of the massage points on the body. For others, you will require a helping hand.

The periosteum has a rich nerve and blood supply. Wherever you massage this tissue, significant changes are generated in the area.

These changes include an increase of blood flow that frequently results in local pain relief. Patients often have good results with chronic pain associated with osteoarthritis, low-back problems, slow-healing ligament injuries, and persistent muscle problems. Acute pain from sprain or athletic injuries also responds well.

As you do this procedure, please keep in mind that osteomassage is not a cure. It is only a simple technique to diminish or alleviate common pain.

I am indebted to Stanley Rosenberg, founder of the Institute for Massage Therapy in Silkeborg, Denmark, for his original help in developing osteomassage and his continuing efforts to refine it. Rosenberg has found that osteomassage also produces a good feeling of deep relaxation within a few minutes, along with increased clarity and energy afterward. At his center in Denmark, and elsewhere in Europe, he has offered short courses in osteomassage to both professionals and laypersons as a form of psychophysical therapy.

"Osteomassage works because it stimulates a mechanism in the nervous system to produce specific, predictable, beneficial effects," he says. "Professionals are generally surprised that osteomassage is so effective and so simple."

osteomassage fundamentals

Where to massage: There are approximately 120 "osteopoints" on the body. I will discuss only those relevant to osteoarthritis pain. You'll be massaging the bony area indicated as an "osteopoint" in the site-specific information below. Work on the bone where the pain is, or if the pain is in a joint, work on the bones that meet in that joint. Osteomassage should not be done on a skin surface injured from a cut, abrasion, contusion (black and blue mark), or any other cause.

Time/frequency: Spend two to five minutes per site two or three times a day, if possible and if comfortable. Do it only once the first day. If multiple joints are involved, start with one or two joints the first day, then gradually increase the number. You may eventually be able to treat all the joints involved at one time if you have enough time and don't become too tired by the treatment. This could take as much as an hour. Don't go beyond that time so as not to become fatigued.

Massage motion: Use small circular motions instead of applying steady downward pressure. These motions stimulate a wider area of the periosteum. You can use the eraser end of a pencil to exert pressure. However, the fingertips are safer and easier. If you find it difficult to maintain finger pressure long enough to complete the massage at a given point, then the eraser tip can be helpful.

The forefinger of the dominant hand is usually the preferred digit, although some people use the middle finger or the thumb. It doesn't make a difference. Use whichever is most comfortable for you as you bring pressure against the bone.

Long fingernails should be trimmed so as not to cut the skin.

Pressure: The amount of pressure applied depends on the physique and condition of the person being treated. It is a good idea to start with light pressure, then gradually increase as you gauge the response.

Apply the pressure downward against the surface of the bone, if that is possible, rather than at an angle.

Always direct the pressure against the bony point. Feel the bone immediately beneath the finger.

Lighter pressure is generally recommended for:

- The first time.
- Pain that is acute or of recent onset, such as after injury. Always be sure there are no underlying fractures.
- Areas of swelling or puffiness around the bone.

- Persons with medical complications, such as heart trouble, lung disease, high blood pressure, or muscle wasting.
- Older persons with delicate bone structure. Heavy pressure for such an individual could cause not only bruising but a bone fracture in certain areas. Take extra care.

Heavier pressure can be applied for:

- Chronic pain problems. They respond better to more pressure than does acute pain. The more acute the pain problem, the less pressure needed to control it.
- People with good bony structures.

A dull, aching sensation, generated by either pressure or massage, is common and frequently indicates that the treatment will be effective. However, any sharp or otherwise unacceptable pain means that you are overstimulating the area. You will still get results, but there is no need to subject yourself or someone else to such discomfort.

Lubricant: It is not necessary to use a lubricant, but it will help in making the small circular motions more effective. Don't use too much. You can use any type of lubricant available in both drugstores and health-food stores. Generally, some inexpensive mineral oil works fine. The choice of a lubricant is not as important as the technique.

Position: It is best to be lying down, comfortable and relaxed, in as natural a position as possible. If that is not possible, sit comfortably in a chair, sofa, or bed. Relaxation is important. The massage should not be done when a person is tense or the muscles are tight due to being in an uncomfortable position.

Stop if you feel worse: Any experience of worsening pain, discomfort, or unusual sensations should be a signal to stop the technique and take a rest. When you try again, if discomfort recurs, discontinue the treatment. Try it again the next day. Sometimes the problem can stem from massaging the wrong location or using an improper circular motion.

massage points

Foot and Ankle Massage

Toes: Arthritis can involve any part of any of the toes. The osteopoints are located on either side of the involved joint or joints.

Ankle: Massage the bony prominences jutting out from the inner and outer sides of the ankle joint. There is another point, located in the instep area of the foot, near the large tendon. Massage the spot where you feel a space between the two bones.

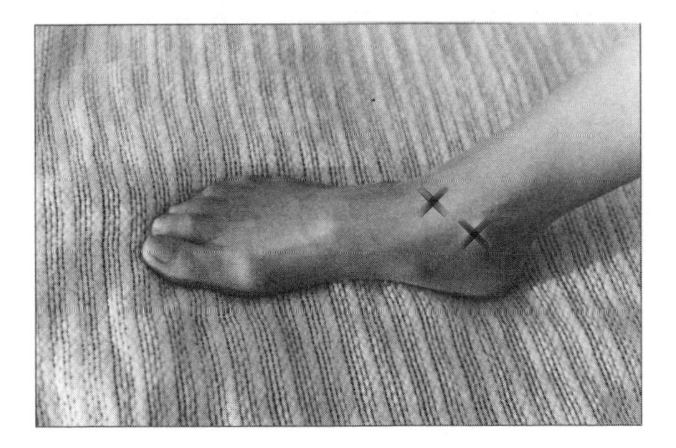

Knee

The primary osteopoint for arthritis can be felt immediately below and to the inside of the kneecap at the ridge where you feel the knee bending.

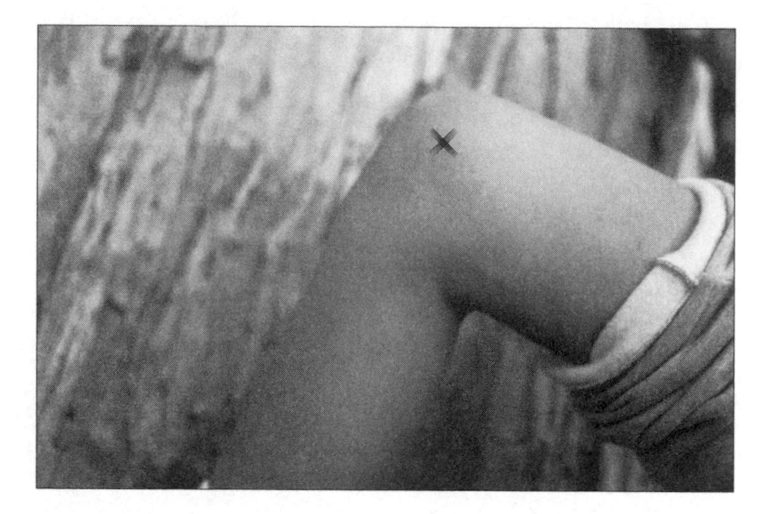

Hip

You'll be massaging the so-called hip point. Treatment is best while lying on the side. Sometimes a pillow placed between the thighs or legs may make it easier to feel the thigh bone. The area is hard to massage but well worth the effort.

Neck

The osteopoints are found along the bottom of the skull bone—one to the left of center, and the other to the right—where the skull joins the neck. These two points are useful for upper neck pain and also headaches that begin at or involve the back of the head. The muscles most affected by stress are attached to these points.

Deep breathing while the points are being massaged can also help relax the neck muscles.

If the pain primarily involves the lower neck, massage the two points located near where the neck joins the upper back. The precise sites are about one inch to the right and left of where the spine "sticks out."

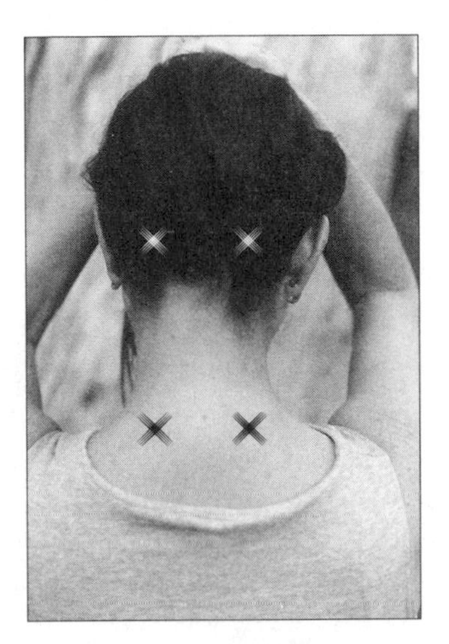

Shoulder

Massage the bony prominence between the end of your collarbone and the armpit. The technique is beneficial not only for arthritic pain but also for recurrent tendinitis and bursitis.

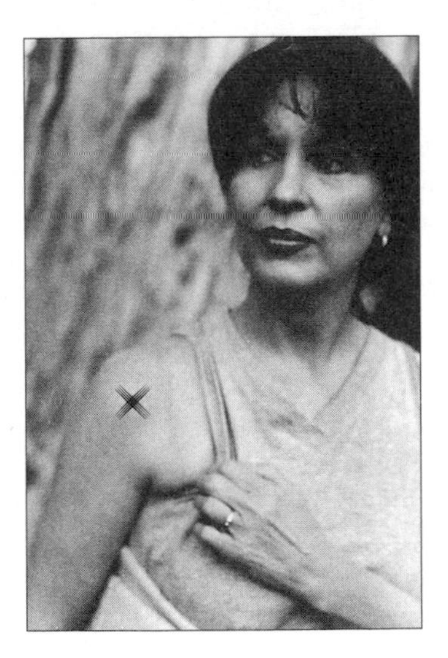

Hands

Massage both sides of any affected finger joint.

The basal joint, a frequent site of osteoarthritis, is located way down at the bottom of the thumb, just above the wrist bone.

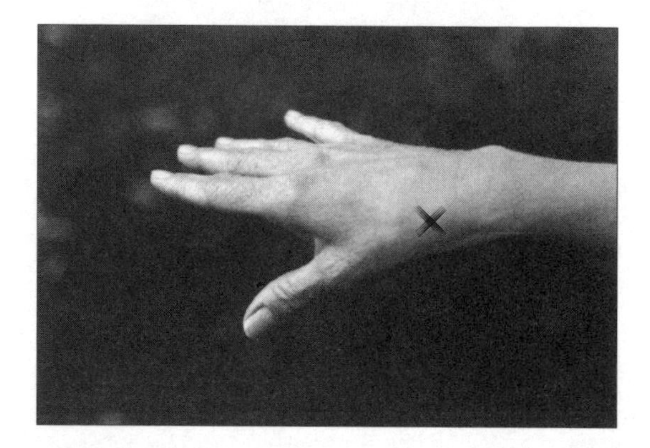

foot care (See chapter 13 on foot care.)

If you have osteoarthritis anywhere from the back on down, I recommend a podiatric evaluation. Arthritic degeneration in the joints of the feet is quite common. This, along with pronation and misalignments of the arches and foot joints, can cause structural imbalances leading to arthritis in the knees, hips, and lower back. So it's wise to have your feet checked out.

Podiatrists will often recommend orthotics. These corrective shoe inserts can help normalize unhealthy foot alignments and also take irregular forces off weight-bearing joints that are bothering you. Redistribution of the weight load in troublesome joints may prevent an arthritic condition from worsening.

Customized orthotics, fitted to your feet by a podiatrist, may cost several hundred dollars or more. You may first want to purchase an inexpensive pair sold at drugstores and running stores. They are often helpful.

magnet therapy

As kids, we all played with magnets and watched with awe as we marched a column of iron filings across a piece of paper by manipulating a dime-store magnet underneath. The same kind of magnetic force is now being applied by increasing numbers of health professionals as a safe (no side effects!) and effective method to help relieve chronic and acute pain and speed the healing process after injury.

I began studying magnet therapy more than ten years ago and have used it in my pain practice to help hundreds of patients, including many arthritics. I have been so impressed with the results that several years ago I collaborated on a book about magnet therapy with Paul J. Rosch, M.D., Ph.D., clinical professor of medicine and psychiatry at New York Medical College. In the book, we summarized the vast amount of scientific research and worldwide clinical experience.

Millions of people use magnets for pain relief and healing purposes. In Japan, China, India, Australia, and Germany, magnets have been popular for many years. In Russia, physicians discovered that the power of magnets was so pronounced that it could reduce the postoperative pain experienced by amputees. Positive studies at respected American universities in recent years have begun to cut into the general skepticism that has long prevailed in the medical profession here. Magnet therapy has been primarily limited to alternative-minded physical therapists, and pain and sports medicine specialists. But today it is attracting a wider circle of medical adherents as researchers validate the benefits for pain relief and healing.

I have spoken to many physicians who routinely use magnet therapy with great effect for patients, including arthritics. Research has shown that magnets applied to affected joints achieve pain reduction in 80 percent of cases. Usually people with pain can expect improvement within a few days to a few weeks.

The precise responses of magnet therapy in the body are complex and not clearly understood. We do know that electrically charged elements—

positive and negative minerals—are attracted to the opposite poles of magnets. This creates a scenario of events inside the body that includes the following:

- increased blood flow and dilation of capillaries
- tissue repair
- reduction of pain impulses
- lessening of muscle spasm
- and the flushing out of biochemical waste products from tissues

There are many different types of therapeutic magnets available, such as shoe insoles, massagers, spot magnets that can be adhered anyplace on the body, and special magnetic wraps for the ankles, knees, wrists, elbows, neck, and back. There are even magnetic pads for arthritic pets to lie on.

For arthritis, I usually suggest mattress pads lined with small, powerful magnets that provide benefits while you sleep. I have conducted measurements of patients who use such pads and have found that they indeed have increased blood flow to the extremities. What could be easier than getting relief while you sleep?

I recommend purchasing a quality pad from a reputable company that will allow you to return the product if you aren't satisfied with the results. One such company is Magnetic Ideas in Sevierville, Tennessee (phone: 800-260-4055; on the Internet at *www.magneticideas.com*). There are a number of other reliable manufacturers making quality products as well. Another is Magnatech Labs, in Palm Desert, California (phone: 800-574-8111; on the Internet at *www.drbakstmagnetics.com*).

If you wear a cardiac pacemaker or any implanted electronic medical device, check with your physician first. And if you are pregnant, it is advisable not to use magnet therapy even though magnets have never been demonstrated to cause problems in pregnancy.

Resources

For more information, read *Magnet Therapy—The Pain Cure Alternative* (Rocklin, CA: Prima Health, 1998), by Paul J. Rosch, Ronald M. Lawrence, and Judith Plowden.

pulsed signal therapy (PST)

In the late 1950s, researchers discovered that bones emit an electrical signal when they are squeezed or compressed. It's a kind of SOS calling for the body to repair, nourish, or otherwise replace damaged tissue. The discovery led to the development of the bone growth simulator, a device that generates pulsed electromagnetic fields to unite fractures that fail to heal within nine months.

Thirty years later, researchers demonstrated in a series of experiments that cartilage tissue also emits a restorative signal when under pressure. They also learned that the signal is impaired in osteoarthritis. These scientific advances inspired biophysicist Richard Markoll, M.D., Ph.D., to develop a device similar to the bone growth simulator that could rescue and restore damaged cartilage. His concept was to reproduce the physiologic signal in the absence of pressure.

Markoll's pioneering work yielded a promising, noninvasive electromagnetic technology that was first tested in laboratory and clinical experiments at Cornell and Yale. The results were consistently and extremely positive. At Yale, for instance, patients suffering from osteoarthritis of the knee, neck, and lumbar spine, received treatments with pulsed electromagnetic signals. They reported major improvements in pain level, range of motion, tenderness of the affected joint, and ability to perform daily tasks. Studies in Canada, France, Italy, and Germany have now produced similar results for more than 100,000 patients.

The patented PST technology is now administered throughout the world for arthritis and sports-type injuries, and, most recently, for temporomandibular joint disorder (TMJ) and tinnitus, not responsive to other therapies. It has even been found effective for periodontal disease. There are more than four hundred clinics in sixteen countries using PST technology. The method is currently approved only for veterinary use in the United States, but approval for application with humans may be granted in the near future. Many Americans have been treated at PST facilities in Mexico, Canada, the Bahamas, and Europe.

I have referred many interested patients to the Vancouver, Canada, clinic where PST is administered. In many cases, the improvement has been remarkable. In the rest, the improvement has been significant enough to allow reduction of medications.

What's more, I have found that patients actually feel better with time. Six to twelve months later they report greater improvement than they did right after treatment.

Here is how PST works: Nine treatments, each lasting an hour, are given daily for nine days. During treatment, patients sit comfortably reading, listening to music, or dozing off, while a pulsed electromagnetic signal is directed to the affected area. The signal mimics the natural emissions of the damaged tissue, activating the healing process and stimulating growth and repair. Studies in Europe have demonstrated that the electromagnetic stimulus significantly enhances chondrocyte and proteoglycan formation in the cartilage, a process impaired in osteoarthritis. The result is enhanced repair of cartilage tissue and restoration of damaged cartilage structures to normal.

Based on the results to date, Markoll strongly believes that PST creates an enduring healing and repair mode in cartilage that has been disrupted by disease, aging, or injury. Moreover, he regards the technology as not just for treatment but "clearly for prevention" as well.

A standard PST series costs about $600, including medical evaluation—a very cost-effective package, in my opinion. There are a variety of other electromagnetic devices frequently referred to as pulsed electromagnetic field therapy, but as far as I know, none of them have the proven research and clinical record of PST.

Physicians who administer this technique are usually orthopedists, orthopedic surgeons, neurologists, or pain specialists.

Resources

For more information on PST or the location of a PST facility, call 888-459-2100, or visit the Internet at *www.pstworld.com* or *www.certifiedpst.com.*

water/heat therapy

I have been a longtime advocate of wet heat to help relieve the symptoms of osteoarthritis and many forms of chronic pain.

Today there are many reusable moist heat packs available on the market that operate either through microwave heating or can be plugged into an electrical outlet. Moist heat is commonly prescribed by physicians for arthritis and other painful conditions. It is preferable to the dry heat generated by heating pads. Dry heat causes a gathering of blood in the capillaries of the skin, whereas moist heat penetrates to a great depth and breadth. This increases circulation throughout the tissue, bringing nutrition and oxygen to joint components and helping to remove waste products in the area. I do not recommend heating pads unless they have a moist heat feature.

Hot tubs (Jacuzzis) also provide relief. If you have access to one, regular soaking helps relax tight muscles and enhance systemic circulation.

And, of course, for a therapeutic getaway, there are always mineral hot springs, prescribed by physicians throughout the ages to help ease painful joints. Today, in Europe, some insurance companies actually reimburse patients who "take the waters." Hot springs and mud packs have a soothing and pain-relieving effect on arthritis. The benefits were recently documented by Israeli researchers. They found that two weeks of spa therapy, including baths and mud packs, produced significant improvement for patients with knee arthritis for up to twenty weeks. The benefits included less night pain, less pain in passive motion, and less tenderness on palpation. Patients needed much less painkilling medication during this time. So, if you have arthritis and haven't made vacation plans yet, here's something to think about.

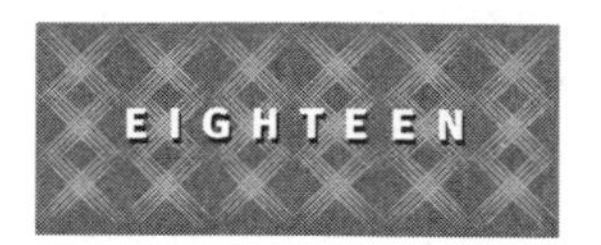

Going the Distance Grandly

I have learned so much from patients in fifty years of treating pain. Among them were many "superpatients," extraordinary human beings—some famous, others not famous—who radiated great humor, joy of life, and the will to overcome suffering. These were individuals who battled pain with spirit, and who brought marvelous survival skills to the marathon run through life. They taught me to age with gusto.

I have treated many people in their eighties, nineties, and even beyond who were active, vital, and passionate. From them I learned that aging is not a disease, it is just a progression in life, and that the fountain of youthfulness is not outside us, but within.

Among them was Beatrice Wood, the famed ceramist, who became a patient very late in her life. Although her hands were filled with arthritic pain, she did not let it slow down her style and zest for life, or extinguish the passion that produced her beautiful pieces of work. She was ever open to new experiences and adventures, even to trying a nutritional supplement called MSM for her pain.

"It has helped a lot," she told me. "I'm glad I tried it instead of some nasty drug."

I vividly recall her 105th birthday celebration in 1998, staged by *Titanic* director James Cameron at the artist's home and studio in Ojai, California. Wood was the inspiration for Rose Calvert, the centenarian heroine in the blockbuster movie.

At the party, someone asked her for the secret of her longevity. "Chocolate and young men," she joked.

A week later, this amazing woman was gone.

Beatrice Wood's art was created not just in her studio, but in the way she lived life. I wish that we all could rise to a similar level of joy. And I hope that this book in some way helps prevent or reduce the pain and limitations that might stand as a barrier.

Good luck on going the distance with healthy joints and all the rest of you.

Scientific References

the osteoarthritis epidemic ahead

Buckwalter, J. A., Lappin, D. "The Disproportionate Impact of Chronic Arthralgia and Arthritis among Women." *Clinical Orthopaedics and Related Research,* March 2000, 372: 159–68.

Cerhan, J. R., et al. "Decreased Survival with Increasing Prevalence of Full-Body, Radiographically Defined Osteoarthritis in Women." *American Journal of Epidemiology,* 1 February 1995, 141 (3): 225–34.

Lawrence, R. C., et al. "Estimates of the Prevalence of Arthritis and Selected Musculoskeletal Disorders in the United States." *Arthritis & Rheumatism,* May 1998, 41 (5): 778–83.

"National Arthritis Action Plan: A Public Health Strategy," The Arthritis Foundation, Association of State and Territorial Health Officials, and the Centers for Disease Control and Prevention, 1999.

Verbrugge, L. M. "Women, Men, and Osteoarthritis." *Arthritis Care and Research,* December 1995, 8 (4): 212.

Yellin, E. "The impact of arthritis: Introduction." *Arthritis Care and Research,* December 1995, 8 (4): 201–202.

———. "The economics of arthritis." In Brandt, K. D., Doherty, M., Lohmander, L. S., editors, *Osteoarthritis* (New York: Oxford University Press, 1998, 23–30).

Yellin, E., Callahan, L. F. "The Economic Cost and Social and Psychological Impact of Musculoskeletal Conditions." *Arthritis & Rheumatism,* 1995, 38 (10): 1351–62.

how osteoarthritis happens

Allison, D. B., et al. "Annual Deaths Attributable to Obesity in the United States." *Journal of the American Medical Association,* 27 October 1999, 282 (16): 1530–38.

Bailey, A. J., Mansell, J. P. "Do Subchondral Bone Changes Exacerbate or Precede Articular Cartilage Destruction in Osteoarthritis of the Elderly?" *Gerontology,* 1997, 43: 296–304.

Chaisson, C. E., et al. "Radiographic Hand Osteoarthritis: Incidence, Patterns, and Influence of Preexisting Disease in a Population-Based Sample." *Journal of Rheumatology,* July 1997, 24 (7): 1337–43.

Chaisson, C. E., et al. "Grip Strength and the Risk of Developing Radiographic Hand Osteoarthritis: Results from the Framingham Study." *Arthritis & Rheumatism,* January 1999, 42 (1): 33–38.

Cheng, Y., et al. "Physical Activity and Self-Reported, Physician-Diagnosed Osteoarthritis: Is Physical Activity a Risk Factor?" *Journal of Clinical Epidemiology,* 1 March 2000, 53 (3): 315–22.

Cicuttini, F. M., Spector, T. D. "Genetics of Osteoarthritis." *Annals of Rheumatoid Disease,* September 1996, 55 (9): 665–67.

Coggon, D., et al. "Occupational Physical Activities and Osteoarthritis of the Knee." *Arthritis & Rheumatism,* July 2000, 43 (7): 1443–49.

Cooper, C., et al. "Occupational Activity and the Risk of Hip Osteoarthritis." *Annals of the Rheumatic Diseases,* September 1996, 55 (9): 680–81.

———. "Individual Risk Factors for Hip Osteoarthritis: Obesity, Hip Injury, and Physical Activity." *American Journal of Epidemiology,* 15 March 1998, 147 (6): 516–22.

———. "Risk factors for the Incidence and Progression of Radiographic Knee Osteoarthritis." *Arthritis & Rheumatism,* May 2000, 43 (5): 995–1000.

Creamer, P., et al. "Factors Associated with Functional Impairment in Symptomatic Knee Osteoarthritis." *Rheumatology,* May 2000, 39 (5): 490–96.

Cvijet, S., et al. "Occupational Physical Demands and Hip Osteoarthritis." *Arhiv Higijenu Rada 1 Toksikologiju* (Zagreb), December 1999, 50 (4): 371–79.

Ding, Z., et al. "National Epidemiological Study on Obesity of Children Aged 0–7 Years in China 1996." *Chung Hua I Hsueh Tsa Chih,* February 1998, 78 (2): 121–23.

Felson, D. T. "The Epidemiology of Knee Osteoarthritis: Results from the Framingham Osteoarthritis Study." *Seminars of Arthritis and Rheumatology,* December 1990, 20 (3 supplement 1): 42–50.

———. "Occupational Physical Demands, Knee Bending, and Knee Osteoarthritis: Results from the Framingham Study." *Journal of Rheumatology,* October 1991, 18 (10): 1587–92.

———. "Does Excess Weight Cause Osteoarthritis and, If So, Why?" *Annals of Rheumatic Diseases,* September 1996, 55 (9): 668–70.

Felson, D. T., Chaisson, C. E. "Understanding the Relationship Between Body Weight and Osteoarthritis." *Baillieres Clinical Rheumatology,* November 1997, 11 (4): 671–81.

Felson, D. T., et al. "The Incidence and Natural History of Knee Osteoarthritis in the Elderly. The Framingham Osteoarthritis Study." *Arthritis & Rheumatism,* October 1995, 38 (10): 1500–1505.

Felson, D. T., et al. "Osteoarthritis: New Insights (NIH Conference)." *Annals of Internal Medicine,* 17 October 2000, 133 (8): 635–46.

Friedrich, M. J. "Steps Toward Understanding Osteoarthritis Will Help Aging Population." *Journal of the American Medical Association,* 15 September 1999, 282 (11): 1023–25.

Gelber, A. C., et al. "Body Mass Index in Young Men and the Risk of Subsequent Knee and Hip Osteoarthritis." *American Journal of Medicine,* December 1999, 107 (6): 4–5.

———. "Joint injury in young adults and risk for subsequent knee and hip osteoarthritis." *Annals of Internal Medicine,* 5 September 2000, 133 (5): 321–28.

Hart, D. J., et al. "Incidence and Risk Factors for Radiographic Knee Osteoarthritis in Middle-Aged Women: The Chingford Study." *Arthritis & Rheumatism,* January 1999, 42 (1): 17–24.

Hochberg, M. C. "Epidemiology and Genetics of Osteoarthritis." *Current Opinions in Rheumatology,* August 1991, 3 (4): 662–68.

Hurley, M. V. "The Role of Muscle Weakness in the Pathogenesis of Osteoarthritis." *Rheumatic Disease Clinics of North America,* May 1999, 25 (2): 283–98.

Keefe, F. J., et al. "The relationship of Gender to Pain, Pain Behavior, and Disability in Osteoarthritis Patients: The Role of Catastrophizing." *Pain,* September 2000, 87 (3): 325–34.

Millender, L. H., Nalebuff, E. A. "Preface to Degenerative Arthritis I." *Hand Clinics,* August 1987, 3 (31): ix.

Mokdad, A. H., et al. "The Spread of the Obesity Epidemic in the United States, 1991–1998." *Journal of the American Medical Association,* 27 October 1999, 282 (16): 1519–23.

Must, A., et al. "The Disease Burden Associated with Overweight and Obesity." *Journal of the American Medical Association,* 27 October 1999, 282 (16): 1523–29.

Nevitt, M. C., et al. "Association of Estrogen Replacement Therapy with the Risk of Osteoarthritis of the Hip in Elderly White Women. Study of Osteoporotic Fractures Research Group." *Archives of Internal Medicine,* 14 October 1996, 156 (18): 2073–80.

Oliveria, S. A., et al. "Body Weight, Body Mass Index, and Incident-Symptomatic Osteoarthritis of the Hand, Hip and Knee." *Epidemiology,* March 1999, 10 (2): 161–66.

Sandmark, H., et al. "Osteoarthrosis of the Knee in Men and Women in Association with Overweight, Smoking, And Hormone Therapy." *Annals of Rheumatology Disease,* March 1999, 58 (3): 151–55.

Sharma, H. *Freedom from Disease: How to Control Free Radicals, a Major Cause of Aging and Disease."* Toronto: Veda Publishing, 1993, 21–25.

Sturmer, T., et al. "Obesity, Overweight, and Patterns of Osteoarthritis: The Ulm Osteoarthritis Study." *Journal of Clinical Epidemiology,* 1 March 2000, 53 (3): 307–13.

Tepper, S., et al. "Factors Associated with Hip Osteoarthritis: Data from the First National Health and Nutrition Examination Survey." *American Journal of Epidemiology,* 15 May 1993, 137 (10): 1081–88.

Van Saase, J. L., et al. "Epidemiology of Osteoarthritis: Zoetermeer Survey: Comparison of Radiological Osteoarthritis in a Dutch Population with That in Ten Other Populations." *Annals of Rheumatology Disease,* April 1989, 48 (4): 271–80.

Wolfe, F., et. al. "Back Pain in Osteoarthritis of the Knee." *Arthritis Care and Research,* October 1996, 9 (5): 376–83.

Zhang, Y., et al. "Estrogen Replacement Therapy and Worsening of Radiographic Knee Osteoarthritis: The Framingham Study." *Arthritis & Rheumatism,* October 1998, 41 (10): 1867–78.

Zwiauer, K. F. "Prevention and Treatment of Overweight and Obesity in Children and Adolescents." *European Journal of Pediatrics,* September 2000, 159 (Supplement 1): S56–68.

the high price of pain relief

American Academy of Orthopedic Surgeons, *AAOS On-line Service.* "Arthroplasty and Total Joint Replacement Procedures: United States 1990 to 1997."

American Medical Association, "Pain Reaches 'Epidemic' Proportions in the U.S," *Science News Updates,* 17 July 1997.

Atkin, P. A., et al. "The Epidemiology of Serious Adverse Drug Reactions Among the Elderly." *Drugs & Aging,* February 1999, 14 (2): 141–52.

Bates, D. W., et al. "Incidence of Adverse Drug Events and Potential Adverse Drug Events." *Journal of the American Medical Association,* 5 July 1995, 274 (1): 29.

Beasley, J. D. *The Impact of Nutrition on the Health of Americans—A Report to the Ford Foundation.* Annandale-on-Hudson, NY: Bard College Center, 1981, 34–36 (Blocking Agents to Nutrients).

Beasley, J. D., and Swift, J. J. *The Kellogg Report: The Impact of Nutrition, Lifestyle, and the Environment on the Health of Americans.* Annandale-on-Hudson, NY: Institute of Health Policy and Practice, Bard College Center, 1989, 298.

Cerhan, J. R., et al. Op. cit.

Cheatum, D. E., et al. "An Endoscopic Study of Gastroduodenal Lesions Induced by Nonsteroidal Anti-Inflammatories. *Clinical Therapeutics,* June 1999, 21 (6): 992–1003.

Fries, J. F., et al. "Toward an Epidemiology of Gastropathy Associated with Nonsteroidal Anti-Inflammatory Drug Use." *Gastroenterology,* 1989, 96: 647–55.

———. "Nonsteroidal Anti-Inflammatory Drug-Associated Gastropathy: Incidence and Risk Factor Models." *American Journal of Medicine,* 1991, 91 (3): 209–12.

Goodkind, M. "Risk of Stomach Bleeding from NSAIDs Varies by Arthritis Type." *Stanford Online Report,* 11 November 1998: 1–3.

Griffin, M. R. "Epidemiology of Nonsteroidal Anti-Inflammatory Drug-Associated Gastrointestinal Injury." *American Journal of Medicine,* 30 March 1998, 104 (3A): 23S-29S.

Johnson, J. A., Bootman, L. "Drug-Related Morbidity And Mortality: A Cost-of-Illness Model." *Archives of Internal Medicine,* 9 October 1995, 155: 1949–64.

Lamberg, L. "Patients in Pain Need Round-the-Clock Care." *Journal of the American Medical Association,* 24 February 1999, 281 (8): 689–90.

Lane, N. E. "Pain Management in Osteoarthritis: The Role of COX-2 Inhibitors." *Journal of Rheumatology,* July 1997, 24 (Supplement 49): 20–24.

Manek, N. J., Lane, N. E. "Osteoarthritis: Current Concepts in Diagnosis and Management." *American Family Physician,* 15 March 2000, 61 (6): 1795–1804.

Moore, T. J., et al. "Time to act on drug safety." *Journal of the American Medical Association,* 1998, 279 (19): 1571–73.

National Sleep Foundation. "Gallup Survey Shows Nighttime Pain Contributes to Significant Sleep Loss for an Estimated One Out of Three Adult Americans." 9 April 1996.

"New Guidelines on Managing Chronic Pain in Older Persons." Medical News and Perspectives, *Journal of the American Medical Association,* 22/29 July 1998.

Osterberg, E. E., et al. "Absorption of Sulfur Compounds During Treatment by Sulfur Baths." *Archives Dermatol Syphilol,* 1929, 20: 156–66.

Page, J., Henry, D. "Consumption of NSAIDs and the Development of Congestive Heart Failure in Elderly Patients: An Underrecognized Public Health Problem." *Archives of Internal Medicine,* 27 March 2000, 160 (6): 777–84.

Pirmohamed, M., and Park, B. K. "The Adverse Effects of Drugs." *Hospital Medicine,* May 1999, 60 (5): 348–52.

Rehman, Q., Lane, N. E. "Getting Control of Osteoarthritis Pain: An Update on Treatment Options." *Postgraduate Medicine,* 1 October 1999, 106 (4): 127–34.

Rainsford, K. D. "Profile and Mechanisms of Gastrointestinal and Other Side Effects of Nonsteroidal Anti-inflammatory Drugs (NSAIDs). *American Journal of Medicine,* December 13, 1999, 107 (6A): 27S–35S.

Shield, M. J. "Anti-Inflammatory Drugs and Their Effects on Cartilage Synthesis and Renal Function." *European Journal of Rheumatoid Inflammation,* 1993, 13: 7–16.

Singh, G. "Recent Considerations in Nonsteroidal Anti-Inflammatory Drug Gastropathy." *American Journal of Medicine,* 27 July 1998, 105 (1B): 31S–38S.

Tibble, J. A., et al. "High Prevalence of NSAID Enteropathy as Shown by a Simple Faecal Test." *Gut,* September 1999, 45 (3): 362–66.

White, T. J., et al. "Counting the Costs of Drug-Related Adverse Events." *Pharmacoeconomics,* May 1999, 15 (5): 445–58.

Wood, A. J., et al. "Making Medicines Safer—The Need for an Independent Drug-Safety Board." *New England Journal of Medicine,* 17 December 1998, 339 (25): 1851–54.

the pandora's box of compounded misery

American Institute for Cancer Research. "Survey Shows Broad Ignorance of Exercise-Cancer Link." Press release, 14 August 1999.

Badley, E. M. "The Impact of Disabling Arthritis." *Arthritis Care and Research,* December 1995, 8 (4): 221–28.

Blair, S. N., et al. "Influences of Cardiorespiratory Fitness and Other Precursors of Cardiovascular Disease and All-Cause Mortality in Men and Women." *Journal of the American Medical Association,* 17 July 1996, 276 (3): 205–10.

Carr, A. J. "Beyond Disability: Measuring the Social and Personal Consequences of Osteoarthritis." *Osteoarthritis Cartilage,* March 1999, 7 (2): 230–38.

Colditz, G. "Economic Costs of Obesity and Inactivity." *Medicine & Science in Sports & Exercise,* November 1999, 31 (11 Supplement): S663–67.

Creamer, P., et al. "The Relationship of Anxiety and Depression with Self-Reported Knee Pain in the Community: Data from the Baltimore Longitudinal Study of Aging." *Arthritis Care Research,* February 1999, 12 (1): 3–7.

Dekker, J., et al. "Exercise Therapy in Patients with Rheumatoid Arthritis and Osteoarthritis: A Review." *Advances in Behavior Research and Therapy,* 1993, 15: 211–38.

DeVane, C. L. "Pharmacokinetic Considerations of Antidepressant Use in the Elderly." *Journal of Clinical Psychiatry,* 1999, 60 (supplement 20): 38–44.

DeVellis, B. "The Psychological Impact of Arthritis: Prevalence of Depression." *Arthritis Care and Research,* December 1995, 8 (4): 284–88.

Downe-Wamboldt, B. "Stress, Emotions, and Coping: A Study of Elderly Women with Osteoarthritis." *Health Care for Women International,* 1991, 12: 85–98.

Elkind, M. S., Sacco, R. L. "Stroke Risk Factors and Stroke Prevention." *Seminars in Neurology,* 1998, 18 (4): 429–40.

Ensrud, K. E., et al. "Correlates of Impaired Function in Older Women." *Journal of the American Geriatrics Society,* May 1994, 42 (5): 481–89.

Guccione, A. A., et al. "The Effects of Specific Medical Conditions on the Functional Limitations of Elders in the Framingham Study." *American Journal of Public Health,* March 1994, 84 (3): 351–58.

Haapala, J., et al. "Remobilzation Does Not Fully Restore Immobilization Induced Articular Cartilage Atrophy." *Clinical Orthopaedics,* May 1999, 362: 218–29.

Hochberg, M. C., et al. "The Contribution of Osteoarthritis to Disability: Preliminary Data from the Women's Health and Aging Study." *Journal of Rheumatology* (Supplement) February 1995, 43: 16–18.

Hughes, S., Dunlop, D. "The Prevalence and Impact of Arthritis in Older Persons." *Arthritis Care and Research,* December 1995, 8 (4): 257–63.

Kampert, J. B., et al. "Physical Activity, Physical Fitness, and All-Cause and Cancer Mortality: A Prospective Study of Men and Women." *Annals of Epidemiology,* September 1996, 6 (5): 452–57.

Lubeck, D. "The Economic Impact of Arthritis." *Arthritis Care and Research,* December 1995, 8 (4): 304–309.

Messier, S. P. "Osteoarthritis of the Knee and Associated Factors of Age and Obesity: Effects on Gait." *Medicine & Science in Sports & Exercise,* December 1994, 26 (12): 1446–52.

Minor, M. A., Lane, N. E. "Recreational Exercise in Arthritis." *Rheumatic Disease Clinics of North America,* August 1996, 22 (3): 563–77.

Oliveria, S. A., et al. "The Association Between Cardiorespiratory Fitness and Prostate Cancer." *Medicine & Science in Sports & Exercise,* January 1996, 28 (1): 97–104.

O'Reilly, S. C., et al. "Knee Pain and Disability in the Nottingham Community: Association with Poor Health Status and Psychological Distress." *British Journal of Rheumatology,* August 1998, 37 (8): 870–73.

Philbin, E. F., et al. "Osteoarthritis As a Determinant of an Adverse Coronary Heart Disease Risk Profile." *Journal of Cardiovascular Risk,* December 1996, 3 (6): 529–33.

Powell, K. E., Blair, S. N. "The Public Health Burdens of Sedentary Living Habits: Theoretical but Realistic Estimates." *Medicine & Science in Sports & Exercise,* July 1994, 26 (7): 851–56.

Ries, M. D., et al. "Relationship between Severity of Gonarthrosis and Cardiovascular Fitness." *Clinical Orthopaedics and Related Research,* April 1995 (313): 169–76.

stop the strains from becoming pains

Buckwalter, J. A. "Osteoarthritis and Articular Cartilage Use, Disuse, and Abuse: Experimental Studies." *Journal of Rheumatology,* February 1995 (Supplement), 43: 13–15.

Cooper, C. "Occupational Activity and the Risk of Osteoarthritis." *Journal of Rheumatology,* February 1995 (Supplement), 43: 10–12.

Cvijet, S., et al. "Occupational Physical Demands and Hip Osteoarthritis." *Arhiv Higijenu Rada i Toksikologiju* (Zagreb), December 1999, 50 (4): 371–79.

Elsner G., et al. "Arthroses of the Finger Joints and Thumb Saddle Joint and Occupationally Related Factors." *Gesundheitswesen,* December 1995, 57 (12): 786–91.

Elson, David T. "Occupational Physical Demands, Knee Bending, and Knee Osteoarthritis: Results from the Framingham Study." *Journal of Rheumatology,* October 1991, 18 (10): 1587–92.

Grandjean, E. *Fitting the Task to the Man.* New York: Taylor & Francis, 1988, 8–13.

Hoppmann, R. A., Reid, R. R. "Musculoskeletal Problems of Performing Artists." *Current Opinion in Rheumatology,* 1995, 7: 147–50.

Jeffery, R. W., French, S. "Epidemic Obesity in the United States: Are Fast Foods and Television Viewing Contributing?" *American Journal of Public Health,* 1998, 88: 277–80.

Newport, M. L. "Upper Extremity Disorders in Women." *Clinical Orthopaedics,* March 2000, 372: 85–94.

Teitz, C. C., Kilcoyne, R. F. "Premature Osteoarthritis in Professional Dancers." *Clinical Journal of Sports Medicine,* October 1998, 8 (4): 255–59.

Van Dijk, C. N., et al. "Degenerative Joint Disease in Female Ballet Dancers." *American Journal of Sports Medicine,* May–June 1995, 23 (3): 295–300.

Vingard, E., et al. "Sports and Osteoarthritis of the Hip: An Epidemiologic Study." *American Journal of Sports Medicine,* March–April 1993, 21 (2): 195–200.

Wahlstedt, K.G., et al. "The Effects of a Change in Work Organization Upon the Work Environment and Musculoskeletal Symptoms among Letter Carriers." *International Journal of Occupational Safety and Ergonomics,* 2000, 6 (2): 237–55.

protect your joints after injury

Biundo, J. J. Jr., et al. "Peripheral Nerve Entrapment, Occupation-Related Syndromes, Sports Injuries, Bursitis, and Soft-Tissue Problems of the Shoulder." *Current Opinions Rheumatology,* March 1995, 7 (2):151–55

Burke, E. "Nutrients Trim Injury Downtime." *Nutrition Science News,* July 1997, 2 (7): 326–30.

Burry, H. C. "Sport, Exercise, and Arthritis." *British Journal of Rheumatology,* October 1987, 26 (5): 386–88.

Cheraskin, E., Ringsdorf, W. M., Jr., and Sisley, E. *The Vitamin C Connection.* New York: Bantam, 1984.

Haederle, M. "Hard Landing—Used to Competing Through Pain, a Former Olympic Gymnast Learns to Live with Osteoarthritis." *People,* 7 August 2000: 131–34.

Kujala, U. M., et al. "Osteoarthritis of Weight-Bearing Joints of Lower Limbs in Former Elite Male Athletes." *British Medical Journal,* 22 January 1994, 308: 231–34.

Lawrence, R. M., et al. "Lignisul MSM (Methylsulfonylmethane) in the Treatment of Acute Athletic Injuries." *Supplement Industry Executive,* March 2000, 4 (2): 37.

Lequesne, M. G., et al. "Sport Practice and Osteoarthritis of the Limbs." *Osteoarthritis Cartilage,* March 1997, 5 (2): 75–86.

Messner, K. "Current Advances in Sports-Related Cartilage Research: Meniscus and Ligament Injuries are Associated with Increased Risk of Knee Joint Arthrosis." *Lakartidningen,* 14 October 1998, 95 (42): 4611–12, 4615.

Roos, H. "Increased Risk of Knee and Hip Arthrosis among Elite Athletes: Lower-Level Exercise and Sports Seem to be Harmless." *Lakartidningen,* 14 October 1998, 95 (42): 4606–10.

Schmid, P. "Whiplash-Associated Disorders." *Schweizer Medizinische Wochenschrift,* 1999, 129: 1368–80.

exercise (but don't abuse) your joints

Blair, S. N., and Cooper, K. H. "Dose of Exercise and Health Benefits." *Archives of Internal Medicine,* 27 January 1997, 157 (2): 153–54.

Buckwalter, J. A., Lane, N. E. "Athletics and Osteoarthritis." *American Journal of Sports Medicine,* November–December 1997, 25 (6): 873–81.

Cheng, Y., et al. "Physical Activity and Self-Reported, Physician-Diagnosed Osteoarthritis: Is Physical Activity a Risk Factor." *Journal of Clinic Epidemiology,*1 March 2000, 53 (3): 315–22.

Felson, D. T., Zhang, Y. "An Update on the Epidemiology of Knee and Hip Osteoarthritis with a View to Prevention." *Arthritis & Rheumatism,* 1998, 41 (8): 1343–55.

Gremion, G., Chantraine, A. "Sports and Arthrosis." *Schweizer Zeitschrift für Sportsmedizin,* November 1990, 38 (3): 13–19.

Hurley, M. V. "Quadriceps Weakness in Osteoarthritis." *Current Opinions in Rheumatology,* May 1998. 10 (3): 246–50.

McAlindon, T. E., et al. "Level of Physical Activity and the Risk of Radiographic and Symptomatic Knee Osteoarthritis in the Elderly: The Framingham Study." *American Journal of Medicine,* February 1999, 106 (2): 151–57.

Miltner, O., et al. "Influence of Isokinetic and Ergometric Exercises on Oxygen Partial-Pressure Measurement in the Human Knee Joint." *Advances in Experimental Medical Biology,* 1997, 411: 183–89.

Minor, M. A., and Lane, N. E. Op. cit.

Panush, R. S. "Does Exercise Cause Arthritis? Long-Term Consequences of Exercise on the Musculoskeletal System." *Rheumatology Disease Clinics of North America,* November 1990, 16 (4): 827–36.

Saxon, L., et al. "Sports Participation, Sports Injuries and Osteoarthritis: Implications for Prevention." *Sports Medicine,* August 1999, 28 (2): 123–35.

Stamford, B. "Cross-Training: Giving Yourself a Whole-Body Workout." *The Physician and Sportsmedicine,* September 1996, 24 (9): 103–104.

eat right and take a load off your joints

Blair, S. N., Brodney, S. "Evidence for Success of Exercise in Weight Loss and Control." *Annals of Internal Medicine,* 1 October 1993, 119 (7 Part 2): 702–706.

———. "Effects of Physical Inactivity and Obesity on Morbidity and Mortality: Current Evidence and Research Issues." *Medicine & Science in Sports & Exercise,* November 1999, 31 (11 Supplement): S646–62.

Burton-Freeman, B. "Dietary Fiber and Energy Regulation." *Journal of Nutrition,* February 2000, 130 (2S Supplement): 272S–75S.

"Element in Diet, Cold Drugs Ruled Unsafe." *Associated Press,* 20 October 2000.

Felson, D. T., et al. "Weight Loss Reduces the Risk for Symptomatic Knee Osteoarthritis in Women: The Framingham Study." *Annals of Internal Medicine,* 1 April 1992, 116 (7): 598–99.

———. "Understanding the Relationship between Body Weight and Osteoarthritis." *Baillieres Clinical Rheumatology,* November 1997, 11 (4): 671–81.

Leermakers, E. A., et al. "Exercise Management of Obesity." *Medical Clinics of North America,* March 2000, 84 (2): 419–40.

Ludwig, D. S. et al. "Dietary Fiber, Weight Gain, and Cardiovascular Disease-Risk Factors in Young Adults." *Journal of the American Medical Association,* 27 October 1999, 282 (16): 1539–46.

Rolls, B. J., Miller, D. L. "Is the Low-Fat Message Giving People License to Eat More? *Journal of the American College of Nutrition,* December 1997, 16 (6): 535–43.

Saris, W. H. "Fit, Fat, and Fat Free: The Metabolic Aspects of Weight Control." *International Journal of Obesity-Related Metabolic Disorders,* August 1998, 22 (Supplement 2): S15–21.

Zitner, A., Cimons, M. "Cold Drug Ingredient Findings a Concern." *Los Angeles Times,* 21 October 2000: A12.

supplement your joints

Booth, B. A., Uitto, J. "Collagen Biosynthesis by Human Skin Fibroblasts. III. The Effects of Ascorbic Acid on Procollagen Production and Prolyl Hydroxylase Activity." *Biochimica Et Biophysica Acta,* 11 June 1981, 675 (1): 117–22.

Cheraskin, E., Ringsdorf, W. M. Jr., and Sisley, E. *The Vitamin C Connection.* New York: Bantam, 1984, 193–94.

Conrozier, T. "Anti-Arthrosis Treatments: Efficacy and Tolerance of Chondroitin Sulfates (CS 4, 6)." *Presse Medicale,* 21 November 1998, 27 (36): 1862–65.

Curtis, C. L., et al. "N-3 Fatty Acids Specifically Modulate Catabolic Factors Involved in Articular Cartilage Degradation." *Journal of Biological Chemistry,* 14 January 2000, 275 (2): 721–24.

Daniel, J. C., et al. "Synthesis of Cartilage Matrix by Mammalian Chondrocytes In Vitro." *Journal of Cell Biology,* December 1984, 99 (6): 1960–69.

Das, A., Hammad, T. A. "Efficacy of a Combination of Glucosamine Hydrochloride, Chondroitin Sulfate and Manganese Ascorbate in the Management of Knee Osteoarthritis." *Osteoarthritis and Cartilage,* 5 September 2000, 8 (5): 343–50.

Deal, C. L., Moskowitz, R. W. "Nutracueticals As Therapeutic Agents in Osteoarthritis: The Role of Glucosamine, Chondroitin Sulfate, and Collagen Hydrolysate." *Rheumatic Disease Clinics of North America,* May 1999, 25 (2): 379–95.

DiPadova, S. "S-Adenyl-Methionine in the Treatment of Osteoarthritis: Review of Clinical Studies." *American Journal of Medicine,* 1987, 83, Supplement 5A: 60–65.

Dovanti, A., et al. "Therapeutic Activity of Oral Glucosamine Sulphate in Osteoarthritis: A Placebo-Controlled Double-Blind Investigation." *Clinical Therapeutics,* 1980, 3: 266–72.

Ellis, J. M., Pamplin, J. *Vitamin B6 Therapy.* Garden City Park, NY: Avery, 1999.

Gaby, A. R. "Are Chondroitin Sulfate and Glucosamine Sulfate Dangerous? *Townsend Letter for Doctors and Patients,* October 2000, 207: 104.

"Glucosamine Sulfate Reduces Progression of Knee Osteoarthritis." *American College of Rheumatology* press release, 15 November 1999.

Greenwood, J., Jr. "On Osteoarthritis, the 'Wear and Tear' Disease . . . Can Vitamin C Help?" *Executive Health,* April 1980, 16: 7.

Helliwell, T. R., et al. "Elemental Analysis of Femoral Bone from Patients with Fractured Neck of Femur or Osteoarthritis." *Bone,* February 1996, 18 (2): 151–57.

Horstman, J. "SAM-e—New Ally in Fight Against Pain and Depression." *Arthritis Today,* January–February 2000.

Jacob, S., Lawrence, R. M., Zucker, M. *The Miracle of MSM: The Natural Solution for Pain.* New York: G. P. Putnam's Sons, 1999, 81–97.

Jonas, W. B., et al. "The Effect of Niacinamide on Osteoarthritis: A Pilot Study." *Inflammation Research,* 45 (7), 1996; 332–34.

Kaufman, W. "The Use of Vitamin Therapy to Reverse Certain Concomitants of Aging." *Journal of the American Geriatrics Society,* 3, 1955; 927–36.

Klenner, F. "Observations on the Dose and Administration of Ascorbic Acid When Employed Beyond the Range of a Vitamin in Human Pathology." *Journal of Applied Nutrition,* 1971, 23: 3–4.

———. "Significance of High Daily Intake of Ascorbic Acid in Preventive Medicine." In *A Physician's Handbook on Orthomolecular Medicine.* NY: Pergamon, 1977, 51.

Lane, N. E., et al. "Serum Vitamin D Levels and Incident Changes of Radiographic Hip Osteoarthritis: A Longitudinal Study. Study of Osteoporotic Fractures Research Group." *Arthritis and Rheumatism,* May 1999, 42 (5): 854–60.

Lawrence, R. M. "Methylsulfonylmethane (MSM): A Double-Blind Study of its use in Degenerative Arthritis." *International Journal of Anti-Aging Medicine,* Summer 1998, 1 (1): 50.

Leffler, C. T., et al. "Glucosamine, Chondroitin, and Manganese Ascorbate for Degenerative Joint Disease of the Knee or Low Back: A Randomized, Double-Blind, Placebo-Controlled Pilot Study." *Military Medicine,* February 1999, 164 (2): 85–91.

Marcolongo, R., et al. "Double-Blind Multicenter Study of the Activity of S-Adenylmethionine in Hip Osteoarthritis." *Current Therapeutic Research,* 1985, 37: 82–94.

McAlindon, T. E., Felson, D. T. "Nutrition: Risk Factors for Osteoarthritis." *Annals of the Rheumatic Diseases,* July 1997, 56 (7): 397–99.

McAlindon, T. E., et al. "Do Antioxidant Micronutrients Protect Against the Development and Progression of Knee Osteoarthritis?" *Arthritis & Rheumatism,* April 1996, 39 (4): 648–56.

McAlindon, T. E., et al. "Relation of Dietary Intake and Serum Levels of Vitamin D to Progression of Osteoarthritis in the Knee Among Participants in the Framingham Study." *Annals of Internal Medicine,* 1 September 1996, 125: 253–59.

Naghii, M. R., Samman, S. "The role of Boron in Nutrition and Metabolism." *Progress in Food Nutrition Sciences,* October–December 1993, 17 (4): 331–49.

Newnham, R. "Agricultural Practices Affect Arthritis." *Nutrition and Health,* 1991, 7 (2): 89–100.

———. "Essentiality of Boron for Healthy Bones and Joints." *Environmental Health Perspectives,* November 1994, Supplement 7: 83–85.

Nielsen, F. H. "The Justification for Providing Dietary Guidance for the Nutritional Intake of Boron." *Biological Trace Mineral Research,* Winter 1998, 66 (1–3): 319–30.

Rizzo, R., "Calcium Sulfur and Zinc Distribution in Normal and Arthritic Articular Equine Cartilage: A Syncrotron Radiation-Induced X-ray Emission Study," *Journal of Experimental Zoology,* September 1995 237 (1): 82–86.

Sangha, O., Stucki, G. "Vitamin E in Therapy of Rheumatic Diseases." *Zeitschrift für Rheumatologie,* August 1998, 57 (4): 207–14.

Schwartz, E. R., et al. "Experimentally Induced Osteoarthritis in Guinea Pigs: Metabolic Responses in Articular Cartilage to Developing Pathology." *Arthritis & Rheumatism,* November 1981, 24 (11): 1345–55.

Seelig, M. S. "Consequences of Magnesium Deficiency on the Enhancement of Stress Reactions; Preventive and Therapeutic Implications" (A Review). *Journal of the American College of Nutrition,* 1994, 13 (5): 429–46.

Shankland, W. E. "The Effects of Glucosamine and Chondroitin Sulfate on

Osteoarthritis of the TMJ: A Preliminary Report of Fifty Patients." *Journal of Craniomandibular Practice,* October 1998, 16 (4): 230–35.

Simopoulos, A. P. "Essential Fatty Acids in Health and Chronic Disease." *American Journal of Clinical Nutrition,* September 1999, 70 (3 supplement): 560S–569S.

Sowers, M., Lachance, L. "Vitamins and Arthritis." *Rheumatic Disease Clinics of North America,* May 1999, 25 (2): 315–33.

Tiku, M. "Evidence Linking Chondrocyte Lipid Peroxidation to Cartilage Matrix Protein Degradation. Possible Role in Cartilage Aging and the Pathogenesis of Osteoarthritis." *Journal of Biological Chemistry,* 30 June 2000, 275 (26): 20069–76.

Travers, R. L., et al. "Boron and Arthritis: The Results of a Double-Blind Pilot Study." *Journal of Nutritional Medicine,* 1990, 1: 127–32.

Verbruggen, G., et al. "Chondroitin Sulfate: Structure/Disease-Modifying Anti-Osteoarthritis Drug in the Treatment of Finger-Joint Osteoarthritis." *Osteoarthritis and Cartilage,* May 1998, 6 (supplement): 37–38.

Weber, P. "The Role of Vitamins in the Prevention of Osteoporosis—A Brief Status Report." *International Journal of Vitamin Nutrition Research,* May 1999, 69 (3): 194–97.

water your thirsty joints

Batmanghelidj, F. "A New and Natural Method of Treatment of Peptic Ulcer Disease." *Journal of Clinical Gastroenterology,* June 1983, 5 (3): 203–205.

———. "Pain: A Need for Paradigm Change." *Anticancer Research,* September–October 1987, 7 (5B): 971–89.

———. *How to Deal with Back Pain & Rheumatoid Joint Pain.* Falls Church, Va.: Global Health Solutions, 1991.

———. *"Your Body's Many Cries for Water."* Falls Church, Va.: Global Health Solutions, 1997.

keep your joints flexible with yoga

Garfinkel, M., et al. "Evaluation of a Yoga-Based Regimen for Treatment of Osteoarthritis of the Hands." *Journal of Rheumatology,* December 1994, 21 (12): 2341–43.

———. "Yoga-Based Intervention for Carpal-Tunnel Syndrome." *Journal of the American Medical Association,* 1998 (280): 1601–1603.

Garfinkel, M., Schumacher, H. R., Jr. "Yoga." *Rheumatic Disease Clinics of North America,* February 2000, 26 (1): 125–32.

protect your hands

Markison, R. E. "Enemies of the Anatomy." *San Francisco Examiner,* 29 March 1998, D1.

Newport, M. L., Op. cit.

foot care—prevention from the ground up

Frey, C. "Foot Health and Shoewear for Women." *Clinical Orthopaedics and Related Research,* March 2000, 372: 32–44.

Gorman, T. "Putting Their Feet Down." *Los Angeles Times,* 13 September 2000, E1.

Subotnick, S. personal communication.

Kerrigan, D. C., et al. "Knee Osteoarthritis and High-Heeled Shoes." *Lancet,* 9 May 1998, 35 (9113): 1399–401.

sex and your joints

Keough, C. *Natural Relief for Arthritis.* Emmaus, PA: Rodale, 1983, 172–73.

putting it together

Buckwalter, J. A., Lappin, D. Op. cit.

doing the extras—acupuncture, chiropractic, massage, rolfing

Berman, B. M., et al. "The Evidence for Acupuncture as a Treatment for Rheumatologic Conditions." *Rheumatic Disease Clinics of North American,* February 2000, 26 (1): 103–15.

Consensus Development Conference Statement on Acupuncture, National Institutes of Health, 2–5 November 1997.

Flechtner, J. J., Brodeur, R. R. "Manual and Manipulation Techniques for Rheumatic Disease." *Rheumatic Disease Clinics of North America,* February 2000, 26 (1): 83–96.

Gottlieb, M. S. "Conservative Management of Spinal Osteoarthritis with Glucosamine Sulfate and Chiropractic Treatment." *Journal of Manipulative and Physiological Therapeutics,* July/August 1997, 20 (6): 400–14.

Zucker, M. *The Veterinarians' Guide to Natural Remedies for Dogs*. New York: Three Rivers, 2000, 62–63.

if you already have arthritis: relieving symptoms and preventing them from getting worse

Blair, S. N., et al. "Physical Fitness and All-Cause Mortality: Prospective Study of Healthy Men and Women." *Journal of the American Medical Association,* 3 November 1989, 262 (17): 2395–2401.

Dekker, J., et al. "Exercise Therapy in Patients with Rheumatoid Arthritis and Osteoarthritis: A Review." *Advances in Behavior Research and Therapy,* 1993, 15: 211–38.

DiCyan, E. *Vitamins in Your Life*. New York: Fireside, 1974.

Doe, D. A. "Medications and Nutrition in the Elderly." *Primary Care,* March 1994, 21 (1): 135–47.

Dryfuss, I. "Exercise May Help Fight Depression." Associated Press, 24 September 2000.

Galloway, M. T., Jokl, P. "Aging Successfully: The Importance of Physical Activity in Maintaining Health and Function." *Journal of the American Academy of Orthopedic Surgery,* January–February 2000, 8 (1): 37–44.

Maibach, E. "On the influence of Japanese Sulfur Baths on Degenerative Arthritis." *Praxis,* 1966, 30: 899–903.

Markoll R. "Pulsed Signal for the Treatment of Osteoarthritis: Double-Blind and Randomized Study Results in Over 50,000 Patients." *Annals of the Rheumatic Diseases,* 2000, 59 (Supplement I): 131.

Messier, S. P., et al. "Long-Term Exercise and its Effect on Balance in Older, Osteoarthritic Adults: Results from the Fitness, Arthritis and Seniors Trial (FAST)." *Journal of the American Geriatrics Society,* February 2000, 48 (2): 131–38.

Minor, M. A., Lane, N. E. Op. cit.

Sullivan, T., et al. "One-Year Follow-up of Patients with Osteoarthritis of the Knee Who Participated in a Program of Supervised Fitness Walking and Supportive Patient Education." *Arthritis Care and Research,* August 1998, 11 (4): 228–33.

Trock, D. H. et al. "A Double-Blind Trial of the Clinical Effects of Pulsed Electromagnetic Fields in Osteoarthritis." *Journal of Rheumatology,* 1993, 20 (3): 456–60.

Wigler, I., et al. "Spa Therapy for Gonarthrosis: A Prospective Study." *Rheumatology International,* 1995, 15 (2): 65–68.

Index